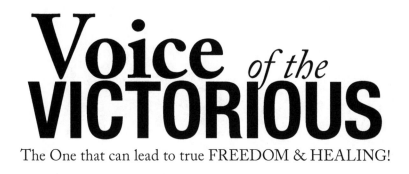

Voice *of the* VICTORIOUS

The One that can lead to true FREEDOM & HEALING!

Sarah Zoe Kainos

WESTBOW
P R E S S®
A DIVISION OF THOMAS NELSON
& ZONDERVAN

WestBow Press books may be ordered through booksellers or by contacting:

WestBow Press
A Division of Thomas Nelson & Zondervan
1663 Liberty Drive
Bloomington, IN 47403
www.westbowpress.com
844-714-3454

ISBN: 978-1-6642-1171-1 (sc)
ISBN: 978-1-6642-1170-4 (e)

Library of Congress Control Number: 2020921800

Print information available on the last page.

WestBow Press rev. date: 11/10/2020

DEDICATION

This is dedicated especially to Dr. "P" and to all those who patiently endured this journey with me and who waged war in the heavenlies on my behalf over and over again. Thank you, Lord JESUS for Your victory, and for giving us a victorious voice! To my family for surrounding me with love and prayers and being willing to share all the Lord has done on our behalf so others could find hope. The Lord God has been our refuge from the beginning and this Psalm of King David has been my life chapter and He has proven it true in me. Maranatha!!!

Psalm 91 (NLT)

1 Whoever dwells in the shelter of the Most High will rest in the shadow of the Almighty.
2 I will say of the LORD, "He is my refuge and my fortress, my God, in whom I trust."
3 Surely, he will save you from the fowler's snare and from the deadly pestilence.
4 He will cover you with his feathers, and under his wings you will find refuge; his faithfulness will be your shield and rampart.
5 You will not fear the terror of night, nor the arrow that flies by day,
6 nor the pestilence that stalks in the darkness, nor the plague that destroys at midday.
7 A thousand may fall at your side, ten thousand at your right hand, but it will not come near you.

8   You will only observe with your eyes and see the punishment of the wicked.

9   If you say, "The LORD is my refuge," and you make the Most High your dwelling,

10 no harm will overtake you; no disaster will come near your tent.

11 For he will command his angels concerning you to guard you in all your ways;

12 they will lift you up in their hands, so that you will not strike your foot against a stone.

13 You will tread on the lion and the cobra; you will trample the great lion and the serpent.

14 "Because he loves me," says the LORD, "I will rescue him; I will protect him, for he acknowledges my name.

15 He will call on me, and I will answer him; I will be with him in trouble, I will deliver him and honor him.

16 With long life I will satisfy him and show him my salvation."

CONTENTS

FOREWORD

This work took almost two plus years to complete. All the drawings within this were part of the author's therapy and are all original. The process was one that caused a tremendous amount of stress and also activated recurring terror dreams once again in the life of the author. The catalyst to finish was knowing that she was called to do it for eternal purposes; to demonstrate that the Lord is God and He is able to heal and renew all that the enemy has sought to destroy. He alone is sovereign and His perfect love casts out fear.

It is this author's prayerful hope that someone may be saved, given hope to breathe one more day and then be encouraged to do the hard work of healing bit by bit, with a trusted professional Christian counselor specializing in complex trauma, and an invaluable prayer team and dedicated godly sponsor.

Be aware that there are parts of this book that can be triggering to those who have been victims of complex trauma or other types of abuse. This should be read being fully cognizant of the fact that you should care for your own heart while working through this memoir of healing.

May you praise the Lord with the author as you recount all that the Lord does on behalf of His children and how He shows compassion to the broken and poor. The work is peppered with several moments of amazing healing and the presence of the Lord and His intimate care for one seemingly insignificant girl, according to the world's standard, from a very rural valley on this earth. You will be washed with the truth of scripture as she was and see that the Lord Who is known in His Holy Word as Jehovah Rapha (The Lord who heals) and Adonai (the Lord of Hosts) has not changed! He still is in the business of being a defender and a redeemer and making the things the enemy meant for evil, work for the good of those who are called by His name and love him!

Pray, read and rejoice!

CHAPTER 1

THE POWER OF VOICES

Growing up in a valley, a literal and figurative one, could be compared to running a modern day spartan race blindfolded and mortally wounded.

This valley was a place where abuse was prevalent yet secret, and in my life, it began as a toddler and continued through early adulthood. To the outsider it was a beautiful place to vacation and get away from it all. Not to those who lived their generation after generation.

This life was also like being in a secret war with fatalities of friendly fire all around. Secret, because you were threatened with excruciating consequences, for yourself and others, if you ever spoke of what was happening to you. Friendly, because the ones that were abusing you and giving you over for abuse, were the ones that were supposed to care for you. Fatal, because you died inside more and more every time it happened, on every level you were silenced.

From my first memories of this life, it is as though each moment I was in a movie which was being directed by a multitude of conflicting voices that demanded allegiance. If you did not obey, there indeed was a penalty to pay.

For this reason, the title of this book "THE VOICE THE VICTORIOUS" was chosen. In time I came to know without a doubt, that GOD alone is able to lead, broken prisoners of dark hopelessness, into freedom and healing. His words can conquer the real enemy. His voice has the only power to completely destroy lies and reveal truth. It has the potential to bring life giving healing to those wounds inflicted on your heart, soul, mind and body.

He uses doctors who love Him in this process of this battle. He is faithful and longsuffering. It is a long-term commitment of each person involved. Many individuals are part of the process, in His service, using their different gifts and abilities, to carry the wounded into victory and wholeness.

Everything can change when in faith you begin and then little by little, healing starts as you intently listen for His voice, believe His promises and let it silence the others.

It is an uphill, slow, grueling journey, traversed a step or half-a-step at a time, so we must listen with discernment and rest often.

FORMATIVE YEARS AND VOICE EFFECTS

In this life, there are numerous different voices we hear daily, continually calling from within and without. This is, in one way or another, the reality for everyone. Voices can either be calming and bring peace or cause you to be overjoyed or they can be vicious and cause you to be frightened. We all are tuned to several voices throughout our lives from the womb to the casket.

As we grow it is clear that the voices, we hear day in, and day out are unconsciously classified mentally and emotionally as either good or bad, calming or frightening and so many other classifications as well.

In an ideal world, the voices of those called to be a child's caregiver would bring peace and joy as well as an expectant excitement when heard by the toddler. Those meant to nurture and care for you should, one would hope, mostly evoke positive reactions and responses.

Unfortunately, today, in the most formative time, those voices bring out the scariest and most negative fight or flight adrenal responses of fear, terror and sadness, warning of impending punishment, abuse, lies, curses, severe pain coupled with isolation and confusion.

Those negative effects were my primary mental, emotional and spiritual reality throughout most of my childhood and teen years. These reactions responses to family members and others stretch as far back as I can remember, to approximately the age of three.

TWISTING TRUTH TO GAIN POWER

Abuse stemmed from everywhere on many levels. Most damaging was the twisting of truth to support the abuse. "No matter what, you must honor your father and mother so that it will go well with you in the land." "Children must obey their parents." were a couple truths that were mutated from the life-giving scriptures to be used to keep me quiet, confused and compliant.

Abuse of power over a child to inflict untold pain either physically, emotionally, and mentally, is absolutely never okay. This type of authority will breed only unhealthy complete dependence on the abuser's point of view and power, as well as untold fear, and shame, allowing the abuser's wicked sense of power and pleasure and control to be kept hidden and ever increasing.

As a young child, I was labeled by relatives on my biological father's side as that one who would shrink back and not like to be touched, who hated to be hugged, or even to have someone sit very close to me. They often would continue to joke about these quirks and mannerisms when I was older. Calling me the different one or the quiet, cold one.

When I began to go to school some of the teachers referred to me as the as the little black cloud. That is what their response was to my quiet, on guard, personality, and what they witnessed on the surface. I functioned out of the egocentric child view of self and new it was not safe to be me.

Inside I would often pretend I felt differently about myself. I would pretend that I was strong, even funny sometimes. In truth, to cope, I always had a running story of what I wished life were like, going on in my mind. Most people were not around to see my safe self-come out, because it would not completely emerge until I was almost 30+ years old. At times a portion of my inside self was shared with those I thought to be somewhat safe: imaginary friends and a cousin who could empathize saw this side of me from time to time.

A SAFE AND HEALING VOICE DOES EXIST ETERNALLY

The voices of abuse and the enemy can only be silenced or translated into truth by the One True Voice of God. His voice is the one true safe and omnipotent Voice and His trumps all others. It can be found in His Holy Word and taught to us through His Holy Spirit and other safe, obedient and genuine servants and shepherds of His Body called the church.

He still uses it to restore and heal. This is what happened to me. Eventually it would completely heal the wounds that I was sure were fatal and had completely shattered me. I still bear the scars and deal with the battle effects, but not alone and not without His presence of refuge and peace. He set me free from the unending enslavement to this valley and those voices of terror and abuse that filled my first 19 years of life.

He gave His life on a cross so that I could have a new redeemed life in Him. It was just a long while before I completely understood and received this in all its power. He never ceased to pursue my wholeness and healing. For that I am eternally grateful and He re-establish my voice in His victory after many long battles for it. I know that He has done this so I will use my voice to speak truth, hope and give praise to His name. May my voice be one that tells the story of His faithful rescue and of His great love. The hope is that others will hear His Voice too and be set free from whatever voices they are battling to silence and overcome so that they may have life. There is great hope, a hope that does not disappoint.

Someone once said that God created us to keep moving forward not backward. That was interesting. If we keep looking over our shoulder at things calling behind us, we will surely run into something or trip over ourselves.

Our eyes are on the front of our head, not the back. We are told that victorious spiritual focus is set on Christ Who is Seated in Heaven, up and forward to our future home. Another part of our body is pointed forward, namely our feet. We use those to walk in a dedicated forward direction most of the time. Spiritually we must also set out to walk in His Steps and they will victoriously lead us Home. Our ears are fashioned to amplify the sound of voices that are in front or beside us. Those voices of both warning and encouragement, so that we can be prompted to move forward toward safety and the next goal, and Spiritually it is listening for the trumpet call of God and that beautiful sound of hope eternal!

Then why does our mind seem to voraciously override this and cling to the power of the voices behind us? Why are they heard so clearly and loudly, as if they were present voices in our faces today?

I believe it is so we remember all that He has saved us from; a trigger of clear warning if we learn to place them in the right category of those that have been defeated and no longer are able to control our thoughts, moods and actions. In remembering, it can also be an aid to stimulate our ability to discern rightly His true voice of truth, power, love and a sound mind; from those voices that would be full of lies, confusion, discouragement and destruction.

That repetition aids in learning is an educational fact. Association aids in mental remembrance. To repeat Scripture, the truth and encouragement of all the teachers, leaders and mentors who have proven themselves safe, true, faithful, and encouraging will strengthen your resolve to live in the present with great hope for the limitless future!

HEBREWS 10:24 (NLT)
"LET US THINK OF WAYS TO MOTIVATE
ONE ANOTHER TO ACTS OF LOVE AND
GOOD WORKS."

By far the best way to eliminate the power of the past is to add to the repetition of Scripture and good voices of truth that can be wielded similar to a shield. One voice when put together with His Voice of Scripture as a sword, then held up higher than the old voices, will conquer them and clarify in your mind that they are now rendered powerless, overcome and taken captive.

Eventually, through much repetition of truth, the power to liberate the damaged mind and heart will be predominant. Then it is free to embrace His voice firmly in all its venues as the One Whose Voice consistently brings courage, strength, healing, freedom and a victorious future! Jesus Christ is the persistent voice of truth and freedom, of healing and the strength to bear up under plodding through healing from repetitive sexual, verbal, physical and mental abuse. He is the voice I had to get ahold of if I was ever to be free, whole, and sane.

THE EFFECTS OF COMPLEX TRAUMA-SHATTERING

The voices that I heard at the beginning of my life were varied in tone and proved to be dangerous and untrustworthy to different degrees. They came from so many different levels of authority and societal power over me that it caused me to retreat often within myself and truly cut off the real world as if the things that were physically happening were not happening to me but to someone else. I have read that the brain of a small child cannot process the severe trauma that is occurring the brain seems to have some choices to make on how to handle these things. Some of the following could be the process it chooses:

1. The brain splits and compartmentalizes the instance. It segregates the moment from reality and categorizes the trauma to a freeze frame of time and to someone else. Essentially telling self that the abuse or trauma is happening to someone else entirely. In this way the small child or individual puts it out of their present memory and then does not need to deal with the physical, emotional, and mental horrific effects at that time.
2. The trauma can presently and profoundly negative impact the persons physical body and this leaves the abused in the present, visibly mentally ill.
3. Then there is a tragic possibility that the trauma is far too great for the child's brain and body and it has no choice but to totally shut down. This could happen literally and the person dies from the severe trauma.

The first choice of these three listed above, is what happened to my brain and physical body. In my brain I created another identity for this to happen to instead of myself.

This was the effect of what is now called complex trauma and ritualistic abuse. The result is also at times called disassociation. A term that struck terror itself in me when I was diagnosed. There is no easy answer or path to dealing with the abuse or the memories.

I would later become well versed in this diagnosis and seek for ways to hurry the healing on in my own efforts. Which only made things harder. Shame, fear, anger and hopelessness is all that I could express. The truth was that the diagnosis was a pivotal step in my healing journey. Facing the reality of the abuse and the terror of those days, with all the truth and consequences and protections that came with it, was a stepping stone toward wholeness.

I sketched a drawing for my doctor during therapy that depicted how it appeared inside to me of how my brain worked. It was like a large open building with many separate rooms off the center. In the center was Jesus and would be ever present with all of my parts. It was a way to set each new identity off from the others and keep it safe in its own room. Cut off from the other ones!

When this was happening, I had no idea that this was what my brain was doing. I was too small to understand or recognize loss of time or new identities. I only knew that things would go black, or time seemed to stop.

The sexual and physical abuse events were so horrific and happened repeatedly throughout my young childhood into young adulthood, that this was the only way I stayed sane and functional daily. The doctor said that it was a gift for coping through such terrible trauma. It also kept me safe from additional trauma as I could hide in the high functioning personality when doing school, sports or youth.

On the hill, in the quarry, the pasture, barn and house - I would go away in my mind and close off from the unspeakable acts and excruciating feelings, all those evil and harmful voices were placed in separate rooms. The real world was disassociated and in this way I could, without knowing, keep it from hurting so deeply or to make it not real, thus detaching myself from it.

This was my only safe and foolproof coping mechanism at this young age and for years to come. In the future it would take years, decades actually, to deal with the effects of all the repeated complex trauma and ritualistic abuse events that I endured. A tremendous amount of repetitive encouragement, that I was now safe and not where those people were at, was needed. I had to come to the point where I could reluctantly allow someone inside those rooms of my brain that had the knowledge and wisdom to safely deal with those paralyzing memories.

All those early years of different levels of abuse and multiple abusers would haunt me at in my young adult years to the point of being unable to function. At night I relived it all over again in terror dreams or during the waking hours, it was as if I was physically there in the midst of it again in the form of vivid debilitating flashbacks.

The dreams still occur now and then; even after years of therapy and the divine supernatural healing of the Lord, and the Holy Spirit's filling and renewing. They are a part of my total memory and like anyone else who has childhood memories, they always will be there. But now they no longer hold the power of rendering me mute, stopping time or causing me to internalize life. I am grateful that the flashbacks have ceased completely now, and I Praise God.

LIFE IN THE VALLEY

The area of the country where I grew up was very rural. Our house was situated between two farms. We lived on what would be considered a small farm along a small creek with chickens, a horse and a large garden, orchard, vineyard, and greenhouse. We kept cows in the neighbor's pastures because they had more room.

We worked on our neighbors' dairy farms. A typical year was putting up hay, trimming trees in the orchard, butchering, making syrup and cutting wood for the winter. There also were daily chores that consumed much of my young daytime hours. School was a welcome respite. I loved it, it was my escape and my favorite place to be. It was this way for a long time, the only true safe place that I had in my life.

In this area hardly anyone went to college. Families stayed in the same houses or on the same land. Generation after generation of the same history were repeated. The same voices of bondage and depression, poverty and hopelessness remained.

Some people went about an hour or further to work in factories in the nearest city, which was in the adjoining state. Some worked in the two factories in the small town about two to three miles away from our house. Most families were farmers or mechanics or general laborers. It seemed as if everyone continued doing what their family did from one generation to the next unless they went into the military.

Few native valley dwellers ever went to college and completed it. In our immediate family as in most, they never permanently moved out of The Valley. Outsiders were not welcome in either. If you were not from there you were considered a threat. We were told not to talk with those people and usually they did not stay around long.

ABUSIVE MATRIARCHAL EFFECT

Our family was run from a matriarchal hierarchy. This sounds like I am writing about a different country in the 1800's. It was only half a century ago. This lifestyle in some areas today is still common. There seemed to be a lot of accidental deaths. There is a high percentage of domestic abuse and abandonment of kids and mothers, resulting in a great deal of single parent homes in this area.

The first voices in anyone's life are those of their immediate family.

Grandmother was the main decision maker as was her mother before her. Mother was the next voice of authority. These were the loudest voices in my life as a child.

For the first five years of my life, my immediate family was made up of two half siblings (each with a different father), my biological father (involved in a secret society and of a very high rank, who became an alcoholic) and mother.

She herself was from a severely broken home with an abusive mother and stepfather and multiple men in and out of her childhood home. Therefore, she was also very damaged by generational ties and involvement in several forms of the occult. I can only hope that she came to truly receive the forgiveness of Christ Jesus and His gift of salvation before she died.

My mother and grandmother purposefully drew my father away from his wife and two sons. Shortly thereafter I was born out of wedlock.

One of my father's sons who lived with his mother was involved in a tragic accident that killed him instantly at the age of 10. I never really knew them; however, I did meet the surviving half-brother after college at my father's house. It was like meeting a repair man. We shook hands and said our greeting then I left and never saw him again.

OTHER FAMILY VOICES

There were many aunts, uncles, and cousins on my father's side, but I did not really know them. There were aunts, uncles, and cousins on my mother's side, who would be a part of changing the course of my life by divine interruption!

My cousin who was closest to me in age and proximity spent a lot of time riding bike and comparing beating stories and talk about how to get out of The Valley! Our lives would be different somehow, and school was our answer. The teachers and coaches that we each had, helped to make that hope a reality, especially for my cousin, who was able to get a full scholarship to a big university far away from The Valley. As far as I know he never returned after graduating, securing a great career and I think even marrying.

TEACHERS AND GOALS

My teachers always encouraged me to be at school and involved in as many things as possible, so that I would not have to be at home as much. One even allowed me to spend a great deal of time cleaning the gym, offices, weight room and basically be a gopher in the athletic department. In return I was able to enjoy the safety of the building and her presence.

Each of the coaches and teachers and other adults were influential people in this small-town society. Unfortunately, some of them also were a part of a group that was unsafe. They were frequently in our home or up on the hill at the quarry where unspeakable things happened.

The voices of those individuals held worldly authority and were both powerful and dangerous to me. I wonder if they realized that they were only pawns themselves of the Father of Lies and evil. The evil beings and horrible things which they summoned and thought they controlled, in reality controlled them.

People that owned these voices were physically older, bigger, and stronger than any child. I was only one of many children that endured such abuse at their hands. Many of the abusers were most likely abused themselves, thus perpetuating the cycle.

The ones that were repetitive abusers in my life are all now dead or in jail. Effects of their abuse caused me to become extremely fearful and wary of people who I interacted with later in life. These people never hurt or abused me but my reactions to them came from a deep-seated real fear and history of severe trauma. If not for the moving of the hand of God itself on my life and His grace and cleansing work to set me free, thus giving me the power to forgive and heal layer after layer, I would have succumbed to their voices and ended my life.

I WAS MARKED AS DIFFERENT: HALF SIBLINGS

As a child in this family I was considered the black sheep for a couple of reasons. I had a different father from my older sister, and she and I both had a different father than our oldest brother. I also was born with, a uniquely different personality, little and the youngest. But, like some younger sisters I really wanted my older brother to like me. I wanted him to be my hero and he ended up being just the opposite.

Because of their clear hatred for me, I would go outside by myself as much as possible. I had my imaginary friends that I would play with on the hill, in the creek and pasture and even board games.

REPEATEDLY ABUSED

One of the times that I had gone down to the pasture to play at the creek and pond. I was walking in the diversion ditch and my half-brother and his friends followed or found me. They then proceeded to abuse me sexually and physically. I retreated into my mind and it was if reality disappeared and all that was happening blacked out and time stopped.

It would happen again and again. One of the most painful memories of this type of abuse happening to me was when I was about 7 years old and some of Mother's distant cousins were visiting. All the adults were in the gully drinking, smoking and carousing. The older kids that were there jumped out from behind an old tree stump in the pasture where I was headed to the creek to play by myself.

The oldest one, who scared me before in the house and that had been harassing me earlier, grabbed me around the throat. Like a wrestler choke hold. He and the others with him, dragged me down to the deep ditch just below the old tree in the center of the pasture where no one could see.

He and the others began to take my clothes off and he pushed me to the ground into the mud at the base of the tree and the rivulet that ran to the creek. They all got on top of me and pinned my shoulders to the ground with one of the boys at my head and their knees pressing into my shoulders. The bigger meaner one that had grabbed me around the neck started to rape me and hurt me terribly. I could not breathe or scream and it hurt so badly. He was so much bigger than I was, there was no way that I could have been able to fight and push him off.

My half-brother was there, and I thought he would rescue me and help me get away from the others. He did not do anything I had hoped for, instead it was as if he was laughing and had set me up and joined in their torture of me. In the middle of it all, I was knocked out. My half-brother was grabbing me by the neck with both hands and pushing hard at the base of my skull in a weird way; while another was there with their hands over my mouth until all went cold and black.

I do not know how much time passed the next thing I remember that day was it being night time and that I woke up in the ditch all muddy and bloody and began crying as I walked to the house.

Mother yelled at me for crying and being a mess. She tore off the rest of my clothes that were all muddy and dirty and spanked me with a leather strap. She put me in an extremely hot tub of water and dumped that same water over my head. Mother kept yelling and cursing the whole time.

All the while she was cursing and smelled of strong alcohol, smoke, and dirt. I stopped crying and everything went black. I went inside my mind where it was safe; where this was not happening, and where I was alone.

Her voice now has been silenced by the soft quiet whisper of my Jesus.

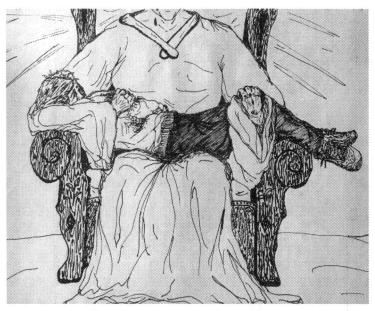

Figure 2-Safe in The Savior's Arms

Jesus cares for us and carries us through the deepest pain inflicted by others and never is too tired to keep us in His everlasting arms!

CHAPTER 2
VOICE OF DADDY

By every appearance he was a man's man. He smoked a pipe, carried a stainless-steel lighter that he would flip back and forth in his fingers on the table all the time. He filled his pipe with sweet apple or cherry tobacco. His pipe collection was amazing, and he had an extensive antique tool collection. He loved to work with his hands. He was a master woodworker, like his father and his father before him. They were all fine craftsman of wood, steel, and the land. They could truly make anything. He was a mechanic and taught mechanics in the evening at the local high school. He was big and handsome and smelled like his aftershave and pipe tobacco and grease.

I loved my Dad! I still love my Dad, and some days I wish he were here to see how I turned out. I hope that he would be proud of me; I think he might be. I can fix almost anything, I try at least, and I love to learn how things work. I have always worked diligently and enjoy a fine car.

He never would say much, but he had a great laugh when he was in the garage with my uncle or talking to my grandfather in the wood shop. He was a good man broken down by the battle of the life he chose.

GRANDMOTHER'S CHOICE AND HIS PENALTY

Grandmother hand picked him for mother's next husband, and father of her final child. It did not matter to grandmother that he was married with two small boys. Immorality or infidelity was not even an issue in their minds. She had seen him one evening in her swinging crystal or an incantation.

I was told this when I was much older by my Aunt, my mother's sister, and oldest sibling. This is how the passing down of the generational secrets worked. It went to the youngest female from my understanding.

I cannot fathom that any of them had any real idea what they were dealing with or what evil they were allowing to control them, it was their way of life, all the evil and the harm they inflicted on those around them seemed to go unnoticed by the outside world.

My biological father did not seem as if he was involved in many, if any decisions in the family as far as I can remember. Mother would call Grandmother about everything. She was the final say in the homelife decisions.

Our family line from grandmother's side lived this way for untold generations in The Valley. Even so, God is greater than the plans of the evil one. What the enemy intended for evil, God can and did use it for good. Praise His Holy Name!!! I am glad He is Omnipotent! He has no rival. She did not and does not have the last say in anyone's life.

HE TURNS TO WHISKEY

Looking back, it appeared that he was too overwhelmed with the life he had gotten himself into. Her wild living and verbal, as well as physical abuse kept him impotent, and unable to make a decision or disagree with her. He resigned to just work, cut wood, fix cars and or anything that broke, and drink whiskey.

He changed greatly after I started to go to school. He began to drink whiskey every night after work. He would sit by the fire in his chair with a big glass full until he was fast asleep. He began to whip me like mother did with the leather straps as well as branches from the closest tree when I would mess up. Messing up would be leaving a tool out, forgetting to turn off the hose, accidentally spilling the small wheelbarrow of wood, or dumping ashes on the porch when I was taking them to the garbage pile outback. I think he was just so angry. I reminded him of the bad choice he made, so it came out in excessive spankings and beatings.

Grandmother at some point turned on him and wanted to get rid of him. She told mother that he was useless and was in the way and holding her back.

I remember waking to loud violent fights where mother would chase him down the hallway with a cast iron pan screaming obscenities and talking in bursts of wicked and unintelligible voices, they were oozing with evil, and it changed her entire being as well as her voice.

Mother and he had more and more fights and then the next while for days I got the brunt of both of their anger. I would try to run away or hide in the shop, doghouse, barn, closet, creek, sluice pipe or anywhere I could get away. The whipping with the leather strap or horse whip or nearest branch was bound to come. Then thrown in bed and the door locked with nothing to eat or drink until sometime the next day when they had cooled off.

The day he left for good, he said that he never was supposed to be my father. He was not cut out to be a parent and he needed to just get away. He threw a glass beer bottle across the kitchen. It smashed on the wall beside the trashcan where I was standing. He walked out the front door, got in his truck and left. He was seeing someone else and finally met and married another.

I stood there with my dog at my feet crying over and over, "I am sorry...I am so sorry...please don't go!" It did not matter how much he would beat me, when he was mad at mother or when he was drunk or angry with his life.

It was at this point that the father of lies firmly planted the lie that I was worthless, a failure, trouble, ugly and unlovable. My own daddy no longer wanted to be with me. I so wished for years and years that he would have taken me with him.

I finally figured out that he would not come back to take me with him. I was now left all alone to fight off all the big people by myself. When he left, my world got much darker and I felt like there was no real person who liked me or would ever genuinely care for me.

I believe he was a victim just as I was on many levels. I see that now. In some ways a victim of circumstance and his own poor choices. But none the less, as an adult he should have stopped the things that went on. Either he was powerless to do so, or he tried and was abused himself for it. I do not know. Nor will I ever know.

In light of all this, one thing that I held onto even in my anger and silence is the fact that despite his leaving me, I truly loved my Dad. When he and I would go on the hill cutting wood, I would ride in the wood truck standing beside him on the front bench seat, like I was the prize trophy he just won at the fair. He would let me work with him in the barn on motors and hand him the tools that he needed. He let me sit on the tractor while he did the work around the house, garden, and adjoining fields.

I loved him and when he was not drunk, he seemed like he loved me too. When we would go up on the hill to cut wood, he used to play this 8-track tape about a daughter being the center of his world. To this day if I hear that song or any words from that song, my eyes well up with tears of sorrow and loss. His voice was one that could make my heart leap to hear it when he was happy and sober...or~ it could make my heart sink with fear and sadness when he was angry and drunk.

After college, I was there for a brief time and I reached out to reconnect with him. Actually, before I came back, I had written a letter to him. He had remarried and was living the life that he always wanted. He was enjoying retirement and travel.

I was glad he had found a new love and was making a new life for himself. I wished him only the best and wished so very much that he would trust Jesus for everything.

He said that he had read of my academic and athletic accolades in the local paper when I was younger. He also said that he was at the plays, games, and the parades. He tried several times to visit me in the hospital when I was in "accident after accident". Each time he was turned away by the staff that said mother had ordered them not to allow him to see me.

He regretted leaving me there, he said he tried to fight for custody, but the judge, lawyer and child counsel were all part of mother's close-knit group. She had worked for a law firm when she was younger as a secretary and they were all close friends at that time. He said he did not have a chance. That gave less power to the years of feeling abandoned and rejected. When I became a parent the fact that he really did not care enough to fight for me was exacerbated.

He could not save me from everything that was to come. Although for years I blamed him for leaving me alone in that situation and escaping himself. Now that I am older and have gone through years of therapy; I know that he too was overwhelmed by what he had gotten himself into. He reacted out of fear, cowardice and blindness to truth.

Because of his involvement with a secret society, it made me extremely nervous and cautious when I was there for any length of time. His voice faded away shortly after this time as he moved far away, and my life once again changed for the worst for a time. He chose once again his own comfort and charmed way of life, over facing truth. I chose not to engage in the secret society and their ways, and it made a deep chasm that could not be broached humanly speaking.

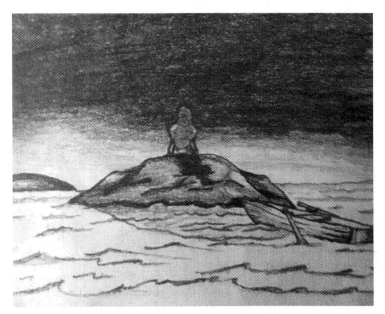

Figure 3-Alone in the Sea of Trauma

I felt intensely alone, unlovable and abandoned. My heart longed for the love of a Godly father and a heart free of fear or trauma. That seemed impossible to ever have.

1 John 4:18(NLT)
"Such love has no fear because perfect love expels all fear. If we are afraid, it is for fear of punishment, and this shows that we have not fully experienced His perfect love."

Psalm 118:6 (NLT)
"The LORD is my helper, so I will have no fear. What can mere people do to me?"

Hebrews 13:6 (NLT)
"So, we can say with confidence, 'The LORD is my helper, so I will have no fear. What can mere man do to me?'"

Isaiah 43:13 (NLT)
"From eternity to eternity I AM GOD. No one can snatch anyone out of my hand. No one can UNDO WHAT I HAVE DONE."

I pray that he came to truly know the Lord as his savior and that he is resting peacefully now that his time here is through. I loved him deeply and he left me when he was in a rage and I did not see him again for months, then not for years, then decades and now never. He has passed away. He died before I could reconcile with him. For that I am deeply sad and regret not pursuing it earlier.

In a different world he would never have left, and I would have been safe. Or if he had left and had fought harder for me then things may have been different. Maybe the first 18+ years would not have been a scene from an R rated movie. A movie that would continue to loop through my brain and hold me captive for years.

Until the time that Jesus my Only Savior, would set me completely free and cut the film and put in a new disc.

Psalm 68:5 (NLT)
"He is a father to the fatherless, defender of widows—-this is God, whose dwelling place is holy."

CHAPTER 3
VOICE OF MOTHER & THE WARLOCK

t is so difficult to even type this. In some ways I feel like I have dishonored and betrayed her in my healing. I know that sounds bizarre to some people. But those who have walked a similar journey will totally understand. When someone who was supposed to nurture and care for you is the one who not only does not fulfill that position, but actively harms, allows/causes, and orchestrates abuse and pain; your brain kind of implodes.

How at the age of near 50 does the thought of her still make me tremble a bit and my blood pressure to go up, shows the extent of the power of her voice. It was one to be obeyed immediately or else, it was one that was louder than all the others, it was one that could use scripture to support evil and it was one that caused confusion that would stump Sherlock Holmes on his best day.

EFFECTS OF VOICES OF THE OCCULT

Because of the powerful ties and influence of the occult in their lives, Grandmother and Mother said they would always know where I was. They had conjured demonic attachments to me that would report back to them where I was and what I was doing. No matter where I was, whether in the woods or by the creek or up on the hill or riding bike; they were there. They would be in my room, and in the barn, everywhere I was they were. There was nowhere I went that they did not go.

Now, most children have harmless imaginary friends that they grow out of. These are a product of being lonely and highly creative. I had one of those that went away as I grew up.

The other "imaginary" friends had voices and were just as powerful as the real humans that surrounded me. But they were demons: frightful, big and evil.

Mother had evoked and directed them to watch my every move and to navigate me to do whatever she deemed best. They would terrify me, and I could not get away from them. Before you write this off as mental illness and something of myth or ancient times. Let me assure you that the spiritual realm is as real as the physical. God Almighty has no rival, Jesus the Son is LORD of Lords, the HOLY SPIRIT is greater than anything of this world. This is truth. Nothing or no one can go toe to toe with Him.

But the fact is that angels and the enemy former arch angel Lucifer or Satan are created beings and absolutely powerful and real and his fallen angels they are limited by God's Sovereign Holy Hand though. Their time is shorter by the day.

These were beings of the enemy. They were not made from my childhood imagination. They were and are figments of evil and they were and are because of the fall and a curse that mother chose. In other countries this is not so abstract. For other cultures, this type of activity is commonplace, but not here in the "civilized" continent.

At least that is the perception. The very real terror they inflicted upon my daily life, attempted sleep and waking thought life is beyond explanation. Do not be overwhelmed by these facts. Do take to this truth to heart, that they did not nor do they ever have the last say. The Lord made sure that those voices, in the end, were completely silenced, thoroughly conquered and rendered powerless by Jesus Himself and His shed atoning blood.

The steps to this victory did not come until I was in my late twenties and at the end of my rope with no hope of ever coming to a place of healing in my limited frontal view.

GENERATIONAL TRAUMA FUELS ABUSE

Mother, must have herself suffered terribly at the hands of wicked abusers as retold by my aunt. Grandmother had passed down the worst of inheritances and it proved that throughout her growing up years, she was in many ways a refined product of her debauchery filled, immoral and wicked childhood home environment.

She ended up choosing the same as grandmother as she got older and then twisted and abused the very thing that could have and was meant to change her life, the WORD OF GOD, as a weapon to enforce even greater harm and abuse. She chose false power and perceived authority and worldly knowledge of the occult over healing, freedom and change.

She allowed men and women in and out of our house and her bedroom like a revolving door. These people from all walks of life would meet on the hill and in the house. They would have seances and plain old parties where alcohol and sex and everything else was rampant. She would quote Indian sayings while in a trance and in different voices, she would have the occult meetings in the kitchen late at night, where they would channel and call the dead, she would use all sorts of new age techniques and often do writings while in a trance. She and grandmother would use a crystal pendant to make choices and decide what or who should be contacted or disciplined. The more she sought it out, the darker and meaner her voice and her life became.

There were those who were the echoes of her voice. The multiple men and women that would be in and out of our house from the time even before Dad left and then like a revolving door after. Some of them would be there for a day; some for months and some for years. They were not farmers and just locals, some of them wore guns, badges, some of them wore suits, some of them came from other places. They looked different then the people of the valley and they acted as if they were friends and to be trusted ~ when you knew deep inside that they were going to hurt you.

WARLOCK COMES TO LIVE

It was never safe when they were there. I would often run up the creek, hide in diversion ditches, in tunnels and in the woods to try to avoid the inevitable. The worst of all these people was the warlock that came to live with us. There was a place in the back of my closet that I could hide that saved me from that warlock. As I think back it must have been my Lord's mighty protective angels that covered me and did not let him find me that night. Because just two rows of blankets and clothes should not have stopped him or hid me. But, that night they did.

From the time she saw him in a trance and then before her as a "spirit" in the kitchen she was completely enthralled with him. Like the way that the Uncle in (Lewis, May 5, 1955)[1] C.S. Lewis classic 6th published novel, "The Magician's Nephew", was enthralled with the evil queen Jadis. That was mother with the warlock who called himself "wizard". He came the first time as an actual human to live with her when I was in sixth grade. He had been around in the woods and in the quarry and other places but until then he did not live in the house.

Whatever he said, she did. He was much younger than she and yet it was as if he had lived a lot longer than her. He would say things that sounded like ancient philosophers and he would draw intensely graphic charcoal demonic scenes and burn incense and chant in some unknown language to me. He was a human, he was just a human controlled by evil, lust, drugs, alcohol and power.

He would get so high and full of evil then he would come after me. I had a wooden door that had slats in it and he would try to pry it open with a machete that he carried and repeated tell me that he gets whatever and whomever he wants. No one can stop him, and no one had the power to keep him away. There literally are years I lived like this. My siblings were older and had moved out and I was alone with just them.

I was a constant target of abuse and yet they controlled me as well. I would defend them and argue with anyone who would say anything against them. The older I got the more that I was full of rage and shame and confusion.

I immersed myself in school, sports, work, and biking. I had a constant battle raging within my mind and heart. I wanted to excel so well that then I could get away, but the need to stay and defend them was just as strong! Literally good and evil vying for my very soul and life. Could I ever be good enough and truly excel at something well enough to please the ones that had the control of my future? I must be the best at whatever was given me to do. There was no room for mediocre or a B. It made me feel as if I had some control in my out of control world.

The wizard became a megaphone of mother's voice and vice versa. His voice was so deep and coercive and smooth that it could make people do whatever he said. He was not a pleasant person whatsoever. If you saw him today like he was then you may think he was a very tall Indian brave from years gone by. He even wore leather from deer he killed, skinned and tanned, tooled and stitched himself. He would walk around barefoot most of the time. Then one day he left to go in the service and they got married and life continued in the downward spiral of confusion, drunkenness, drugs, alcohol and debauchery and mother turned to women as partners in this evil life as well.

She would have women in the house that lived with her and that were abusive. She was always one to defend them and tell me to get over it and that now she loved them. As if she even knew the meaning of that word. I awoke one night when both my siblings had long since moved out and there was this strange women and mother on top of me holding me down and abusing me. When I screamed, she simply told me it was for my own good, that I had to learn to play the part that she played. She clamped her hand offer my mouth and everything went black.

EFFECTS OF THE VOICES OF POVERTY

For a time after Dad left, we were quite poor. We stood in line to get cheese, powdered milk, bread and peanut butter with black and white labels in town at the fire company. We put up a lot of vegetables from the garden, had chickens that gave us our eggs, the dairy farm we worked on gave us milk and we helped with the butchering. I had my own steers and we also had an orchard, so we had apples and pears and grapes when they were in season. We had a root cellar that we dug out in the side of the hill that held the apples, potatoes and carrots that got us through the winter months. There also was deer season where we would get deer and can the meat to have the meat all year long.

That time of tremendous poverty served as a catalyst that drove her deeper into evil and want of power and the riches of the world. She craved something she could not reach no matter what avenue she chose. No amount of men, women, evil or syncretism could make her complete. She was deceived and she then chose to inflict the same harm on others and eventually things spiraled out of her control and that which she thought she controlled, really controlled and turned on her.

Mother was increasingly becoming more arrogant and blatant in her immorality. She went back to university and gained a high position that paid well for the area. She was keen in worldly knowledge, extremely intelligent and used her executive position in a hospital to gain some sense of inflated worth in the town where it was located. But, in the small town where we lived no one could see her any differently though. Her reputation was set.

Even with her working there it seemed like we did not have money for the basic things.

I worked at the nearby farms, from the time I was 9-10 years old, to earn money for my school clothes, coat and shoes and anything else I needed for school or wanted to eat. It was by working for them that I got my dogs. They had farm dogs and when they had pups, we could choose one if we worked for them. I learned so much being poor. I learned the value of hard work and planning and trades that I have been able to help others with now. God uses everything for our good and His glory. One day. One day in the future. Perseverance is the key to overcoming the tribulations of this world.

When I got older and later in high school, she would come in my room and say that I scared her (figuratively). I was too quiet; I was thinking too much and not telling her what I was thinking. I knew people she did not know and spent too much time reading. She could no longer tell what I was thinking and although it unnerved her it actually gave me some hope. That in my mind was indeed the safest place to go. She could not read my mind. I would go there often from that time on, and continue to get quieter and quieter when around her or anytime I had to be at the house.

MOTHER ATTEMPTS TO END HER LIFE

One night someone came to the school to pick me up from play practice, I was in the orchestra and I usually biked to grandmothers and then went with mother whenever she would pick me up. This night was different. Mother was in the hospital that she worked at in the psychiatric unit with an attempted suicide and overdose. It had caught up to her and she was overcome. Grandmother was stone cold and said that it was nothing to cry about that mother was weak. This would make her stronger and it would not happen again. It never did. She indeed seemed to get harder from that point on and yet more manipulative around me.

A few months later I awoke with mother over me again. I said I just had a dream with Satan telling me I was going to burn, and that mother had given me to him and that she was a fiery witch. She said, simply. "Oh, that is what you think? Well, it is true. My name is means fiery witch."

No rebuttal, no argument at all. Cold, curt words of simple fact. As far as she was concerned, I was something to be used, manipulated, controlled and hammered on until she could conform me to herself. It would make me stronger, more powerful and self-reliant. It would form me into her. It formed something horrible in me that is for sure. Something that only the blood of Jesus and His authority, years of relentless therapy and a dedicated prayer team, learning the power and truth of the Word of God and speaking that truth in the places where lies and evil were resident could redeem.

During those years of ritualistic abuse, sexual abuse, verbal, emotional and mental abuse I became so fragmented. There were times when I would lose days and there were times when I was not sure how I ended up some place. It was frightening to say the least. I would compartmentalize those times and put them away in my brain as if they were not happening to me. At so many points after these years, I truly did not know who I was or why I even existed. I was a walking shattered window of stained glass, with only the fragile outside edges holding me together.

The adults around me were not helpful. They did not stop or report the abuse. The teachers in high school that knew about it only said they were sorry. They wished there were more they could do. Honestly, I think they feared mother and grandmother and did not want to "get involved" with that kind of stuff. Back then I do not think there were any laws in place to make them accountable to the knowledge that they had. Like so many others I am sure that it was easier to look the other way and hope for the best. Thankfully, that is not allowed today. If a teacher or other authority figure knows of abuse, they are required to report it.

HOPE AMID THE DARKEST EVIL

The time when a friend invited me to her youth group, and I saw a different type of adult and people that I had never seen before shook my world. Everything would begin to turn in a different direction and a new path was being bushwhacked for my freedom and for a new life for me from that point on.

Praise be to God! He had something so much better than another generation of evil. He would completely change my direction and my inheritance to one of His healing, redemption, cleansing, freedom. It would come in time.

He grieves at the trauma inflicted on children, on all people. His vengeance on the evil one will be full and complete. Jesus conquered the enemy and he is rendered powerless in the lives of His redeemed children. He is the Lamb of God that took away the sins of the world, He is the conquering King that conquered death, the grave and hades. He is the Lord of Lords and no one will take away those that are His and His alone!

One friend from the youth group, had me move in with her after mother's suicide attempt, for several months. But that did not last long. I was summoned to go back to the house, and I obeyed mother. There was still a hold she had on me and when she would say certain words, I had to obey. I did not have the strength of soul, heart or mind to fight it.

I also had another friend that tried to stand up to the warlock and he was much younger and had no idea who he was dealing with or that it was so unsafe for him to even get that close. We ended up driving two hours away to get away from the warlock after that episode, so that he would not brutalize him. The warlock followed us for so long and at last he ended up turning around when we got closer to where his parents and other Christians were staying at a retreat center.

I spent a lot of time running away and hiding when the warlock came back from the service. I was his prime target as well as that of mother and her cohorts, they abused me out of hatred. Because when he was away in the service, I had heard about the real God Almighty and His Son Jesus and the Living Word.

That friend that had invited me to her youth group where I heard the gospel and saw a people that were so vastly different than anyone one from the valley. I had committed to living my life differently for Him and would be baptized (at the angst, outright anger and protests of mother) there in that place.

That choice, stirred up more trouble for me than honestly, I could handle at that age, and I was always in a battle with them from that time forward. I was finding it hard to live and wanted to escape any chance I could. They now knew I would not be like mother; I would not follow in her footsteps. They were livid!

STANGERS IN THE VALLEY WERE MY SANCTUARY

None of the people in that forbidden church were originally from the area and you could tell. The place was off limits to me for as long as I could remember. Every time we would drive by it or several homes of the people that went there, I was told they were a cult and would brainwash me into believing something that would make my life much worse. It was as they say, "The pot calling the kettle black." When I was healthy and free and remembered this is sounded so ridiculous! The truth was just the opposite of what I was told.

But hind sight is always clearer. Your vision is often blurred when you brought up with evil being called good and wrong being portrayed as right. That is why scripture says that it is foolish to compare yourself with yourself. You must look to the Lord Jesus

Christ as the standard and His Word and the source of truth and rules for Holy living.

I would try to go to the youth leaders' home as often as I could after school, by bike or car. I would just sit and watch them live their lives out and wonder how this could be real. I did not have to talk or engage with them. I was just being in this bubble it seemed. They were so kind and loving to their kids and their clients and each other as a husband and wife. I sat in awe and had so many questions going on through my head. They were an anomaly to me.

It never mattered what time or route I would take to get to their home, I was always caught sooner or later. Often times when I would bike there, just as I got their grandmother would call their home and tell them I was not allowed to be there and send me back immediately. I could never adequately explain how this happened. It happened throughout my life as I was hundreds of miles away in places, they would have no knowledge of. They would either call that place and ask to speak to me and or someone would end up being there to bring me back.

There would be no escape except for a Christian college or death. I did not know how I could ever afford college, and your parents must sign. I would work my tail off to get the best grades and get a scholarship. But even then, it was not enough. Two separate attempts at going to University ended in me returning to only a worse situation and no money.

He and mother's voices were the last and hardest ones to silence. In the final stages of healing they were completely replaced by The Redeemer Himself, King Jesus and the sound of a doctor who loved Jesus and desired to see healing and wholeness brought about by the Holy Spirit and Jesus shed blood on the cross. Only when these two voices and the fear they evoked were destroyed, could I clearly hear the voice of the Lord Jesus and the truth of His Word and receive freedom and healing.

All the other voices that were there at her command could

be silenced a thousand times easier and years sooner than that of hers.

The blood of Jesus Christ and the persistence of His servants to be obedient and faithful in their work as His hands and feet here on this earth. Would need to time and again remind me, some days it seemed like it was continually, who I am in Christ Jesus and the truth of what His Word says about Him and about His children.

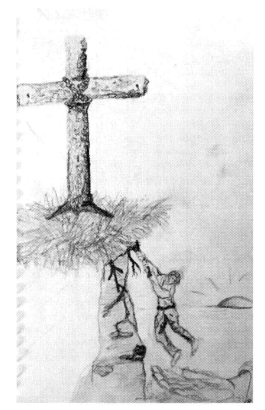

Figure 4-Stop Striving & Let Go-He has you!

When we feel as if we have no more strength to hold on to the only source of hope we have~ relax and let go of your striving~ His outstretched hand is beneath you and He will catch you!

CHAPTER 4
VOICES OF FLICKERS OF LIGHT

There are always points of light that we do not see until we look back into the darkness and see those twinkling stars. My Aunt, the CEF director, some teachers, the youth leaders, the pastor at that forbidden congregation and the friend that first invited me to go, were all bursts of light and His loving hand.

After my Dad left, my Aunt took me to a summer day camp to get me out of mother's way for a while. In this day camp I met someone who would change my life both for now and all eternity. My Aunt came to know the Lord a lot later in life and she had no one to disciple her in the faith or teach her systematic theology, but she loved me and tried her best to make life more bearable for us kids.

The camp organizer was an older lady who noticed me moping around and asked me to sit down beside her on a bench. My Aunt had filled her in on my home life and she asked if I wanted to meet someone who loved me and would never hurt me or ever leave me? I quietly said, looking down at the ground and kicking my feet at the dirt, that I did. (I can remember it like I am still sitting there that summer day) She introduced me to Jesus, God's Son and His promise to be with me forever, no matter how dark and scary it might get. He would never ever leave me once He came to be my friend.

I owe an eternal debt of gratitude to both my Aunt and that faithful servant to rural backwoods kids who needed to hear the gospel and have some kind of hope of a better life, one free of abuse, abandonment, oppression and fear.

From that time on I would often hear a still whisper in the darkest scariest times saying, "I will never leave you. It will get very dark, but I will never leave you." But it was clear, and real and in time proven to be absolutely true. Even though at the time it certainly did not feel like it.

If it were not for God's gracious intervention in this small life, I would not be here. I would also be separated for all eternity from Him Who created me a masterpiece for good and not for evil. This was one of many times that He intervened to save me from myself as well as others and the evil one.

RELEASE TIME A CALLING FROM THE LORD

Matthew 19:14(NLT)
"Let the little children come unto me. For such is the Kingdom of Heaven."
- JESUS

They continued to have what was called "release time", with that same director, after school began, once a week. My aunt made sure that I was to be there. She would come to the school and walk myself and several other children across that small town to the meeting place. We would sing and learn about this Jesus and His coming again to take us home to heaven in the clouds. The song went something like a rocket countdown and I can see the big songbook that looked like an old rocket with clouds around it. Oh, that sounded good. But as a small child it did not seem like this would ever be a reality for me. That was just like a movie on tv; the time would come to an end and we would walk back to school, and I would have to go to the home that I lived in here on earth. That was just the opposite of something to look forward to or good.

I was given a Bible by my aunt and attended a church that was fine on the outside. But inside it had the some of the same people that would twist the truth, use evil and abuse to get their way and cause harm. The area was full of generational sin and strongholds of the enemy. This building was no different, it was just a building of stone and wood. When mother would get angry with me, which was most of the time, she would call me either my aunt's name or my dad's name, and say I was just like them.

Thankfully, most of those people have since died that filled that building. But, my Aunt, she meant well and wanted to help me find hope. She was a light and safe harbor and I have fond memories of her and how she made the unbearable-bearable.

The CEF director resigned and moved away. Years later, when I got older and had a driver's license, I looked for her to ask her some more questions and see what she knew. She was no longer in the area, the lady that had taken over for her said she "burnt out". At the time I had no idea what she meant. I can only imagine the battles she fought there. She needed encouragement and support that was not available. But she had a part in changing this life. I will always remember her and thank the Lord for her and my Aunt's love and willingness to come alongside a child who was broken and withdrawn and in desperate need of some kind of hope of safety.

There was another light in my childhood. It was a fourth-grade teacher that confronted mother about my intense quietness. She and the other grade schoolteachers had nicknamed me the "Little Dark Cloud". Like from the childhood story of the little dark rain cloud. All the tests I took in school had showed that I knew all the material and that I was gifted, but I would not speak unless coerced to answer a question.

She was not afraid of mother; I could tell as I sat at the small desk in front of hers with my head on my hands. She stood about a head taller than mother talking with her face to face. I would later come to find out that she was a believer in Jesus Christ and was a member of the forbidden church that would be a transition to freedom one day for me.

A SAFE HARBOR COMING INTO VIEW

Lighthouses were coming in the way of the one who invited me to a youth group and the leaders that were in charge for years to come.

These lights were powerful while living in the darkness day in and day out. I was in middle school when my best friend at the time, who knew that my life was awful kept asking me to come with her to her church youth events.

Even though she herself was not allowed to come home with me or go places with me, nor were any of my "friends" permitted, to stay at my house. (When we were older, they came for the alcohol and everything else they were not supposed to have at their age.) But, when we were younger, and their parents had a say in where they went and with whom. I was off limits. My house was off limits. It was known. It was a small town.

But, despite all that, she invited me to a youth group at her church. The one that was forbidden, for those of us who grew up generation after generation in the valley, to go to.

I said that I would not be allowed to go. She said to ask if I could go with her to a group thing for the kids in class. Her family would pick me up. Amazingly enough, I could go. Mother knew the father and said that he would make sure I was home when he said I would be.

Well, when I walked into that church it was like nothing I had ever seen before. The people were different than the ones in my life sphere. You could tell they were not from around there. At least their families had not lived there for generations. They talked a little different and the leaders of the youth group had this look of joy in their eyes. Like they really liked the kids and they were believing what they were telling us. They seemed so kind. I was so drawn to them, but inside I was repelled at the same time. I wanted what they had. I wanted what those kids that were there had. It was completely different. Words cannot fully explain how opposite it was to anything I had ever experienced!

Little did I know that this was another hammer blow on the chain of bondage, the Lord would use all these moments to set me free. This was stepping out into unknown waters, risking the wrath of mother and grandmother. Making my own choices and receiving the blessings and consequences from those decisions. I was growing up and being drawn by His Hand of Grace and Mercy to Himself. He was calling and reminding me of WHO HE WAS and IS. The adventure was going to get more exciting and dangerous.

THE PRICE TO PAY FOR STEPPING AWAY FROM EVIL

Every time I went to a youth event there was always screaming and other physical beatings as prices to pay for being with "those" people. One specific time we had an event that was to be an overnight at a campground where several Christian artists were to perform. I was very reluctant to go and did not want to "sleep" near anyone.

In the middle of the night I was walking with the leaders and my best friend back to our site and all of a sudden it felt like someone was strangling me and then I could no longer see and blacked out. I awoke in an ambulance on the way to some rural hospital emergency room in another state. I tried to escape as all I could see were strange men over top of me putting tubes in my nose. I panicked and they gave me a shot.

Then I woke up in a bed in the ER with the youth leader who was my best friend's mom standing there talking with the doctors. They said I had some kind of a seizure and blacked out. I could not bring myself to tell them that someone was choking me, and the evil voices were cursing and that I continued to hear them as I lay there in the bed. I figured I was going to lose my mind and I did not want these people to shun me. So, I said nothing. I took their medicine and they released me and sent me back to the campground where one of the older helpers drove me home in my car the next day.

When we arrived at the house, mother was livid that I was at this event and furious that I went to a hospital. She grilled me about everything they asked me and what I said and if they did any tests. I was kept from going to youth group for several months after that. She said that if I ever told them anything about our family, she would make sure that I would not be able to speak ever again. She was wrong. There were temporary silences, but He is more than a conqueror on my behalf.

Praise be to Jesus who gives us the victory! He gives me a voice of triumph and praise to my God for all He has done and will do! All this has happened so that I would not rely on myself, like the Apostle Paul, but that it would be only by the power of God and His mighty hand that I would press on and be set free and live as an instrument in His hand of healing and peace.

As a teenager your friends are what define you and your place in society as a whole. This does not change tremendously when you mature, but it is key as a youth. I tended to be a loner for safety sake. Let us just be clear. Kids can be extremely cruel. If we look deeper into why they are cruel it is often because hurt people, hurt people too. In our area there was a lot of poverty and a lot of hurt. Those that were well off were few and far between, but they definitely let you know who they were and that what they wanted or said was all that mattered. I believed it.

So, when they would say that I was ugly, or was a bother or that, most likely I was, never going to be anything or was going to be just like my mother, I believed them. Although I was intelligent and athletic, I had books and sports to make me feel better about myself, I was not pretty, wealthy or from a normal family. In response to all the things they would say, notes they would leave in my locker or in a book or on a chalkboard I went deeper within myself.

ETERNAL HEART CHANGES ONE NEW YEAR'S EVE

There was one friend who was younger than myself who tried to encourage me to not listen to them to be my own person, he was the son of the youth leaders. Again, so different from the other families of the area. At first, I shrugged him off as a pipsqueak and just wanting to be friends with an older kid. He obviously wanted something other than just to hang out with me. In time he proved to be a true friend that wanted the best for me, even if I did not know what that was or who that was. He did.

This friend and the one that invited me to the youth group in the first place also invited me later to a New Year's Eve all night lock-in at the church. This is where they would play volleyball in the youth center and make homemade pizza and tell each other stories until the next morning into the New Year. He said that his parents and other youth group leaders would be there and even some of the kids that had graduated and went off to college were back and were going to give what he called their "testimonies". I went.

It was a safe harbor, definitely a lot safer to be there than at the house with who knows and all the awful things that would be sure to happen that night. The warlock was now in the service and overseas and we had to go there earlier that year and it ended up with me basically seeing much of the surrounding countries on my own on the Eurail as they did whatever.

Now mother had all her other people at the house, and it was worse than ever. My siblings had long since moved out and one was married and having a baby. She was due three months after they got married. So, the idea of not being at the house and no need to tell mother where I was specifically going because she was otherwise incapacitated, sounded phenomenal. I was driving and had bought my own car with my own money, so that gave me some freedom.

About midnight we were all sitting in one of the classrooms munching on snacks and the older youth leaders were getting pizza ready when one of the college kids started sharing about his life. He said about his parents always fighting and how his dad would favor his older brother and that he felt worthless and was into drinking and doing all sorts of things to numb his feelings of worthlessness. Then he came here and learned that the Lord Jesus did not want him to be perfect before he accepted his gift of forgiveness, that it was a process that the Lord would clean him up once he took the gift of salvation. He said he thought he had nothing to lose and wanted Jesus to be Lord of everything in his life. He then shared about how that changed his hope for his life, that he had a purpose and he never felt alone like the empty feeling he had before. He knew he could not have made the changes that he made in his life without Him.

I will never forget him or how his eyes almost danced as he said the last part of his story and then another college kid began to tell her story. I was mesmerized. Literally watching these older kids that I had no idea who they were, but they were definitely different and they were full of life and laughed and really liked each other.

If this is what it meant to allow Jesus, to whom I was introduced to on that park bench so many years ago, to be Lord and make me clean I wanted that more than anything else. I then thought, there is no way He can make ME clean. If these kids only knew all the things that I have been part of and the awful dirty things that were done to me. I was too broken and dirty and ugly for Jesus to clean me up.

A WAR OF COMPLETE SURRENDER AND HOPE

There was a war that began that evening. A deep powerful war that began to rage. Screams that would pierce your soul and voices that would make your stomach turn began to rise within me. I asked Jesus to be my Lord that night, to please forgive me and make me clean, really clean.

Then my next thought was a plea. Could He take control of these things and voices, the pain and my home life and rescue me and help me to live for Him and get me out of here? It was a cry of desperation. It was heard and His voice began to speak into my life through His Word the Bible that I could not get enough of after that, and through those Youth Leaders, those college kids, my first Christian tape that I bought and hid in my room.

Oh, how that means so much to me now some 30+ years later. That these new voices would battle for me, against the dark voices and the ever-present voice of mother and grandmother and those around them.

I would work very hard mowing lawns, cleaning houses, trimming orchard trees, working at the greenhouse and any other odd job that I could from then on in order to save up money to go to college. I now wanted to go to a Christian College and major in Art and Architecture. The youth leaders said that there was a college that did not require tuition only room and board. I thought that would be perfect. I applied and was accepted.

When I graduated several of those classmates wrote in my yearbook. The resounding theme was that they never thought I would make it alive or they were sure that I would end up being just like my siblings. But, because of the friend who had the courage to invite me to that youth group and show me that there was something different and that Jesus could make a difference even for me the daughter of a witch living in a house of debauchery and evil, I did make it out alive and on to the next chapter of my life.

I visited the university and loved it and its art program was phenomenal. The lifestyle would be a complete change for me. I was a farm kid, athletic and casual. That was not the dress code at this school and in the end, I only lasted 2 weeks. There were several other factors that came into play with my leaving. But I left dejected and sent back to the valley to work another year and try to figure where to go from there. I now was changing dramatically, and the warlock was back from the service and the house was even more of a war zone.

I had begun unashamedly going to the forbidden church. I was 18 now and I also was living with a friend's family for that year because of the warlock and mother. The Lord soon opened another door of escape and I began the process of applying to yet another Christian college. I was accepted and began plans to move. I sold all the belongings and packed up what I had left and set off for this new beginning. New hopeful voices to overshadow the old ones that still haunted me awake or asleep in those days.

CHAPTER 5
VOICES OF DECISION
~ PROFESSORS AND COACH

As I entered the new college the fact that it was small compared to the other one that I had attended previously seemed comforting in a way. Also, this one was much more affordable with the scholarships, grants and financial aid and work study that I had secured to make this a possibility. I would encourage myself mentally that I could do this. The fact that I was now out of the valley, gave me a glimpse of hope that I could begin a normal life, seemingly like everyone else that was shuffling around me. I could pour myself into the studies and become a famous architect and never need the help of anyone ever again.

Somehow my plans for escape and betterment were always turned on their heads and this one would be no different than the other times I tried to get away and become invisible.

The school was in a small suburban town, it was a former orphanage. It certainly was not a challenge to me academically as I had hoped, but it did challenge the voices that lay in wait for me every moment that I would be in a quiet place or close my eyes.

It was far enough away from the valley to not expect that someone would just show up and make a scene. This feature would raise the hope that it would be safe here and I could start living the life that I wanted to live. I could do this. I had joined the volleyball team and that required we be there early. That was perfect. They did not have a band or orchestra. I was a percussionist and the drums were often a great coping mechanism for me when I would feel enraged or scared.

Volleyball would be my outlet and the coach were fierce, tough and demanding. Until volleyball camp I was never able to do a proper pushup. Her commanding us to get down and do it with such authority and intensity pushed one. Not in a negative way. She simply carried an air of respectful authority. At this point I had no idea that the Coach would become a key player in my spiritual freedom, new life and overall growth.

THE DREAM OF BEING AN ARCHITECT DASHED

The art professor was the death of my dreams of becoming an architect. He would put me in the center of the studio with my piece of art pinned up in front and point out every area that was incorrect. He would then ridicule my view of the subject and mock my intended presentations. He turned a passion that was a healthy outlet and my hope of a career into disdain. His voice resounded with those peer's form school that screamed I was ugly, a misfit and would never amount to anything more than mother.

I went to the dean of students and changed my major to physical education and recreational leadership. I would not let him turn my art and that private sanctuary of the sketchbook into something that would cause me pain. I would keep it for myself. I could be a teacher of physical education. I was gifted in athletics and it would be my new focus. The Dean of Students introduced me to my new advisor-COACH! She was so demanding as a coach how could I survive her being my advisor. If I survived the valley, I could take her that was for sure. I already was teaching 9th grade athletics and health during high school because of being an Honor Student with completed academics by my Junior Year. I could do this.

PHYSICAL EDUCATION & SPORTS

Sports became a year-round pursuit. There was not a sport I did not play. Coach would send me to the wall for my attitude several times and she had talked with the dean of women and the dean of students regarding perceived abuse. I was unaware at her astuteness during this time. She was watching me closely and was concerned. She had heard from my roommate that mother had been calling the floor on the pay phone and making me upset. It had become daily, until the roommate had finally begun to tell her that I was not there and make up some excuse.

I was not able to make enough money by doing one work study so I asked for additional work so that I could pay for books and other necessary life items. They granted my request and I began a new work study in the office as an assistant to the secretary to the President of the school. This was God's hand. This would prove to be His way of beginning to open my ears to hear Him directing me into trust. Because I still trusted no one. This also, would be HIs way of creating a path for an entrance into a new spiritual family.

That work study was right outside the office of the coach. The secretary was always dressed like she walked out of a fashion magazine and her makeup was flawless. I had never been around someone of her caliber and it set me on edge. With this office setup it was easier to work for both and do what was expected more efficiently.

There were several professors that year that caused me to take a deep look inside and wonder if I really had the stuff to make it in this life. The dean of women was also the professor of biblical studies and was amazingly intelligent. She spoke with eloquence and insight into scripture that would draw you into the pages. As much as she intimidated me, she also intrigued me. How did she gain such insight, where did she study, what did she read, when did she decided she wanted to pursue academia? Were just a few of the questions her classes provoked.

Professor of Psychology caused me concern. She was always asking questions of me after class, and I would try to be polite and excuse myself without upsetting her. I did not want my grade to suffer because of my need to protect myself. I knew that if anyone here found out what I had come from, or whom my family was I would probably be kicked out. That is what my college kid brain surmised incorrectly. This professor would pick the Coaches brain after practice about me and I happened to walk in on one such session. I was in the front office working and went back to ask Coach when I needed to set up the gym for the basketball game that night. I almost walked directly into this professor as she handed Coach a book for that kid on your team. I was that kid.

THE BREAK THAT CAUSED A BREAKDOWN

Soon Thanksgiving break was here, and I was unaware that you needed to leave campus.

Little did I know that I would have to return. I was sent back as it was required that no students could stay on campus during breaks. It would be a turning point in the process of breaking free.

If only they had known what they were sending me back to. How could they? I did not let on that anything was different from anyone else's background. I was extremely guarded and well versed by now in keeping quiet. I was an athlete and self-sufficient. No one, I thought, at that time other than my roommate had any idea of my life.

I truly had nowhere else I could go. So, I went. It was horrific. When I came back to school, it was after a week of being abused, held at gunpoint by the warlock and threatened that if I walked out that door, I would regret it. I escaped from his grasp and that gun at my temple only by the grace of God. He gave me supernatural strength to beat him with the drumsticks in my hand run for the car and drive as fast and as far away as I could get.

Volleyball players came back a day earlier than other students other to practice. For that I was extremely thankful. I took my stuff up to my room and as I was walking down the hallway to use the restroom one of the other volleyball players came out of her room and innocently said "WELCOME BACK! How was your vacation?". I completely lost it.

I could not speak, I felt like I could not even hear any longer and I ran for my room locked the door and dove into my bed. Sobbing. Sobbing like I had never ever done before. Because I was told you did not cry. If you cried, then you would get hit harder or beat more so you learned to stop crying and just hold your breath. But there was no holding this in any longer.

Well, I completely lost track of time and missed practice because I could not quit crying and could not breathe. I heard a voice at the door, and it was Coach! I was mortified and said I was sick and could not go to practice through the sobs. All of a sudden, the door opened, she let herself in and began to tell me I should really talk to somebody. That they had a counselor on campus that would talk with me and give me choices. I did not need to go back to whatever I came from.

There was no way I could talk to someone. She had no idea what she was asking. I would suck it up and get it together and be at practice the next day. I felt like a complete misfit walking into practice after missing it, with the other teammates asking me if I felt better.

After that practice Coach called me to her office. She sat me down and told me after yesterday the dean of students had arranged for me to talk to a school counselor about my home life. My response was an emphatic NO!!! I did not ask to talk to anyone. I asked her if I had to meet with this person in order to stay in school. She said that it would just be helpful, and that they would just ask me a few questions and give me some suggestions. It would make me a better student and a better player. She framed it in such a way and with her authority it was almost impossible for me to reject the offer. So, she made an appointment the next day in her office.

UNHELPFUL STUDENT INTERNS

That proved to be one of the many times that someone trying to help made it worse. They were not equipped to care for the trauma that I suffered nor the outcome of their prying. This made the rest of the year that much more difficult in way of night terrors, mother's phone calls increased and life in general was more stressful. Her voice became very loud once more, and I would retreat inside my mind again. The difference would be this time, that there were genuinely caring safe people observing this and praying for wisdom in how to best help me. I was simply unaware of their efforts and their prayers at this point in my life.

The end of the semester came, and the school had arranged for me to work at the little Christmas tree stand and store that they had each year to raise funds for the college. That way I would not need to go home and would have a legitimate purpose for staying and working for financial aid.

I was a worker and that was one thing that my upbringing had taught me well. Work hard and often. The people I worked with did not ask why I was there they simply treated me as an employee and paid me each day when I was finished. This made the break go very quickly and the final semester of the first year was soon underway.

CHAPTER 6
VOICES OF THE SUMMER STRANGERS

The local camps in the area came to all the colleges to look for summer help. I was encouraged to apply for one of the summer positions by coach. One of the camps was part of the church where Coach attended. She had invited the whole volleyball team to her church, and we went with some reluctance. It was quite different once again from even the church that I had attended with my youth leaders. It was much bigger and had several pastors not just one. Interesting. The lady that I worked for in the office was also there along with her family. Things were starting to come together in my head. Their voice was one in the same. One of help and encouragement. At least that was their desire.

I was accepted as a camp counselor and began work the week after school was out. This was working out great. The only downside was I would be working in a camp with a cast for the summer as I had shattered my foot during volleyball season but had not let coach take me to the doctor. Then I just taped it for softball season. Finally, when I could hardly walk, she took me to the athletic trainer at another school who then made her take me to the sports medicine clinic. Broken in 5 places. They casted it and said I would be in it for 8-12 weeks because I had waited so long. So, the entire summer of camp counseling would be in a walking cast!

But this too was all part of the Lord's plan for me to have some time to be still and silent before Him without interruption and to draw me out of the valley into freedom. Because I had to go over very early in the morning to the director's residence to use a handicap accessible restroom, I was able to have time to listen to praise music and have time away from the campers and other counselors to regain focus. Because I did not sleep much due to terror dreams and flashbacks, this was a vital gift to carry me through this difficult summer.

The summer was great, and I was busy all the time so I tried to keep the overwhelming voices and memories at bay being busy. But, when you have a cabin full of young campers you cannot be screaming out when you sleep, or they will get scared and ask a lot of questions when they wake you up.

This is exactly what happened during high school camp week. Some of the kids in my cabin were from the youth that I was working with for Christian service. Those high school young ladies on one evening, after lights out, came to the porch steps where I often sat after the campers went to sleep inside the cabin, and asked if they could pray with me. I immediately put up my guard and said that they could pray that I would sleep well and not dream, I sure would appreciate it. We prayed and they went back in and got in their bunks and nothing more was said the rest of the week. The sleep did not get much better but the stress of them knowing was gone.

Those same girls are young Mom's today and it is amazing how the Lord has had them cross my path from time to time and now we are able to rejoice in all that the Lord has accomplished!

Voices of young and innocent strangers were a gift to me as I was hiding in the shadows of past complex trauma. Little encouragements were taken in and treasured. There was a suspicion and fear at first of what they might know and I would replay everything I said in my mind to make sure that I did not reveal anything that might cause me more harm. In the end those small glimpses of light and kindness returned at just the right time to bring hope during darker times in the future.

It is indeed true that random acts of kindness make a significant impact in lives you otherwise would have no interest in except for that brief moment. Brief moments can change eternal moments.

It was that same week that the head counselor from the cabin across the path came over to me in the middle of the night as I sat outside my cabin watching the stars and praying. She just chatted with me and asked me if the kids in my cabin were afraid of the crickets chirping like the kids in her cabin? It seemed so strange to us that such a little noise could cause such fear in kids from the city. Yet loud honking, gunshots, and sirens had no effect on them whatsoever. They hated silence. It is the desensitization and familiarity of a cacophony of constant noise day in and day out. Something different instilled fear. I understood fear.

As we talked, she simply sat down beside me and chatted. She never asked why I sat out there night after night. She never asked about my past or where I was from. She simply was being a friend. These types of encounters would begin happening more and more. It was the Lord's weaving me gently into a new family. A safe family. A healthy, large, amazing and godly family with a heritage of "adopting" others. God was beginning to place me, "the lonely" in a family. It would not be an easy transition for anyone. This young lady would one day marry one of the brothers of the family that would "adopt" me. How the Lord's hand works from day to day in our lives as we look back, is utterly awe inspiring!

Truly the scripture in **Proverbs 16:9** is accurate and proven in our looking back:

"We make our plans, but the Lord determines our steps"
was borne out in my lifetime and again. He is Jehovah
El Shaddai the God Who sees.

At the end of that summer all the counselors, directors, and other camp staff went to the beach for a retreat and a time of debriefing after a long summer with hundreds of campers and situations that arose with each week.

I had not been to the ocean and the beach since I was young with mother and grandmother. That trip was awful. This one would hopefully be better. I wondered what it would be like to be there again since I was only 6 the last time, and it was difficult to remember anything but being sick, burned, the smell of rotten fish and that the milk tasted like the fish smelled. Then there was the added trauma of a hurricane and being left at the motel with my siblings while mother and grandmother went somewhere for a couple of days. This had to be better!

This time it was much different! We had all formed friendships and a counselor bond that summer and were there to encourage each other. There were several evenings of times just sitting, chatting and singing worship songs around a campfire. Lots of laughing and remembering funny camper stories.

One of the great highlights for me was the first time I ever had the privilege of leading a young camper through the salvation steps. They had given us a bracelet with beads on it to help us teach what it meant to be saved by Jesus' sacrifice on the cross. I thought that was an amazing tool. I would never forget that summer and that young camper. I pray that she is still walking with the Lord and being used mightily for His kingdom.

No one even mentioned the night terrors that they had to wake me from nor did any of them ask me questions. I was so thankful. I was anonymous of sorts and not from the area nor their churches.

We headed back to go our separate ways. The retreat ended

with me crashing my car in a surprise flash flood on the way back to the camp! That little car was smashed by a huge station wagon, it went to a junk yard and I went to a hospital in another state with a bad concussion, cuts, bruises and scratches.

Unfortunately, this meant that before school started, I had to go back to the valley...I had to go get another car and get back without getting hurt by the warlock or trapped. When I tried to get a hold of someone to come and pick me up at the director's house no one would.

I finally called my old youth leader in hopes that they could somehow come get me. They said they would be happy to come and get me. I offered to reimburse them for their gas and their time and did not expect them to do it for free. I could not LET them do it for free. There was something in me that feared owing anyone anything! They came and allowed me to pay them for their gas, time and meals. That took a chunk out of the money I earned for being a counselor, but it was well worth it. I was grateful and fearful at the same time. I dreaded going back and what would happen.

The Lord made a way in the desert for me just as He did the Israelites of long ago. An exodus of sorts. This would be the next to the last time I would ever be there. He provided a car that was not being used for $100.00 and made the transition as if I were almost a different individual to everyone. There is no other way to explain it other than God's complete protection over me at that time. Like I had a bodyguard with me or a cloaking device that you see in the science fiction movies.

He has worked on my behalf repeatedly in amazing ways! Even when I felt like I deserved nothing but death, hell and eternal damnation. But He has given me forgiveness, eternal life, grace, mercy, healing, strength upon strength and oh so much more. Praise Him for all He has done and will do until He returns and after!

I have learned that he uses even what the enemy might have

meant for evil, for our good and His glory in the end. Now I had a more reliable car- I thought, and unfortunately, I had it from someone who would want to hold it over me as a controlling issue. I had no other choice other than to buy it from mother. I could not afford anything else and I needed to get back to school as soon as possible. As I headed back to school the brakes went out and I would have to exit the highway by shifting down and letting it coast into a curb in a small-town rest stop. My first thought was that the warlock probably messed with the car before I left, and I was meant to not make it back to school.

Yet, I choose to believe that the Lord allowed that car to break down, and kept me safe, so that I would have something to trade in on a different car one day. A car that myself and others often referred to as, the JESUS CAR. Its name was because it was the only possible reason that it ran for so many years and passed inspection with minimal repairs. I fixed the muffler with a soda can and clamps, the radiator hose with electrical tape and furnace tape and the tires seemed to last forever. Every time it passed inspection; I felt a huge sigh of relief. Like the Israelites shoes in the desert, so was my little beat up car. It was a great conversation starter with the youth as well. Whom many of them learned to drive in the parking lot at church in that old stick shift beat up car.

A new semester and a new year of hope for a better future. If I could get through this year and get a degree than I would be free of the valley and all the horrors of my past. Sometimes the path to get to the other side is through a deep dark valley, and this valley would last a lot longer and be one of the valleys of the shadow of death several times. Not so unlike my childhood shadows, they were still with me. They would rear their ugly heads and I would be paralyzed with fear.

CHAPTER 7

VOICES OF INQUIRY ~ PEERS

Another semester of another year at school began and this time I was asked to be an RA on the floor. This meant an increase in financial aid and the room cost was taken off the bill making it much more affordable. Thank you, Lord, for these small tokens of care and provision. Unfortunately, my best friend and roommate began to ask more questions. She was bolder and more in my face that year.

After about the second full week of volleyball camp when the rest of students were to come back, I was having increased intensity terror dreams and talking and screaming in my sleep. When my eyes closed, I would relive my childhood and the last 18 years every night. No matter how far away I was, it was as if I had never left and they appeared to be right there in that room abusing, beating and chanting evil incantations over me.

It felt as if I could not escape, those evil things that I had lived through as a child were haunting me every night. I was embarrassed and harassed all at the same time. My roommate was not going to let up questioning me until I gave her an answer. One day during her questioning I told her as plainly as I could without giving her any details or names that my life was not the best growing up and unfortunately, I was reliving it every time I went to sleep.

After a few months it would happen during the day and I would lose hours and sometimes days at a time where I could not remember what had happened or what I had missed. I was existing not living. This would increase in frequency in the coming months and years.

My goal became not to sleep when others were around. I would try to stay awake by any means I could. I would study later and later; read, bike, draw, listen to music and monitor the halls and stairwells throughout the night. I would not sleep unless my roommate was out of the room for an extended period of time at class or gone for the weekend. Sleep deprivation was having a huge effect on every aspect of my life. Its results began to be quite evident to the coach, my professors and other staff members that I interacted with for my work study. My health would really begin to suffer not to mention my strength and my feeling of intense aloneness. I began to withdraw once again and go for long walks after class, rain, snow or sleet. I would sit on the edge of bridges contemplating why I was even here. This would begin a downward spiral.

A few weeks later the pay phone at the end of our hall began ringing every evening after dinner. This was a long time before cell phones. Someone would generally answer it if they were close by. It was mother. She would call drunk, or stoned, or just in a trance and telling me that if I did not come back, she would send someone to get me. That I had to be there with her, that I was not like those others in that school. I would listen and tell her I could not that I paid for the school and I was going to complete it. She would say how I was an awful person and a horrible daughter and start yelling and cursing at me and the people walking by could hear it and stare as they walked up the phone. I would hang up and walk away numb. I was becoming known as the kid with the psycho parents.

Truly those girls had no idea what I was dealing with on the other end of that phone, nor what I had dealt with my entire life.

I was sure if they ever really found out, they would tell the Dean of Students and I would no longer be an RA; or worse than being fire, they may even kick me out of their Christian college because I certainly did not belong there with the rest of them and their godly families.

TRYING TO COPE

Walks became drives over to a nearby lake. I would sit on the edge of that lake thinking that I was truly all alone. The walks after class and after practice were longer and longer. In my heart I never wanted to be with others unless necessary ever again. I did not even want to be seen. If only I could be invisible and just do my own thing and not bother anyone else and they do not bother me.

This was impossible, because my mind was replaying over everything more and more and all those screaming voices and evil voices from the valley were growing stronger and stronger and I was growing weaker and weaker. In all aspects, physical, mental, emotional and spiritually as well.

After one particularly loud and traumatic phone call my roommate stopped me and said that she told the other girls that if she called not to tell me and that I never needed to answer that phone again. She made it clear that no one on that floor cared what she said about me or who she was. I ran out of the dorm and she followed me and we walked in silence to the bridge where I would sit and she simply sat there with me for over an hour and I thought and stared at the water rushing under our feet. It looked so inviting.

She said it was time to go back before practice. I knew that practice and hitting that ball with everything churning inside of me would be a particularly good thing. We got up and started the walk back to the gym. On the way back an SUV pulled up beside us and the window rolled down. It was the lady I worked for in the office. She wondered if we would be interested in going with her family to a house they owned in the mountains for the weekend. She had checked with Coach and we did not have a game and I was off for the weekend from monitoring. I said immediately, "No, no thank you." My roommate on the other hand told her we would think about it and let Coach know and she would call her.

CHAPTER 8
VOICES OF CHALLENGE
~ FUTURE FAMILY

A s we walked to the gymnasium, she said she thought it would be good for me to be around that lady and her family. My roommate knew them well as she was older than myself and had been at the school two years longer. Coach agreed with her and said that she was good friends with them and they went to the same church and that if I would look around on Sundays, I would see them serving at the church.

My red flags of self-preservation went up and would remain up the entire weekend. Why would they want to invite college kids to hang out with their family? What did they want from us and where was the house and who all were going to be there? It simply did not seem like a smart thing to go off into the mountains in an area you knew nothing about with strangers! This seemed like an awfully bad decision. It went against everything within me to go. My roommate insisted as did Coach.

After practice, the Coach told me to meet her in her office before, I went to work study. She said that she really did think that I should spend some time with this family. That it would be good for me to see how they live. Just watch them and listen and they would not make me talk if I did not want to. I asked her what they wanted from me. Why would she ask me to go with them unless she wanted me to work for her or something worse?

As I talked, she proceeded to walk out to the administrator's office and tell her I would be going with them. UGH! I was sure that this would be awful. One of the many times I was completely wrong.

I thought that my roommate would be going too, so at least I would have her to hang out with. Then at the last minute my roommate could not go because she was not feeling well. Once again, I felt lured and trapped into a situation out of my control. I was going to be in a car riding with some older woman I did not know up to an unknown location somewhere in the ambiguous "mountains". Sounded like the beginning of a great murder mystery. Like much of my life.

That Friday night she pulled in student parking and jumped out of the car all cheerful and asked if we were ready to have a great weekend away. Then my roommate told her she would not be going because she was sick and handed her my duffle bag. The others that were supposed to be riding with us were not in the car and she could see that I was panicked. She told me on the way to her home that the others were already up at her mothers-in-law house and we would be meeting them and her sister-in-law.

When we pulled in her house my heart sank as I saw this incredibly tall man with a beard on the roof with their daughter knocking down an old chimney. He looked enormous from where I sat, and I told her I would wait in the car. My insides felt as if they all just melted and my worst fears were about to be realized. I was wrong again.

After she gathered the things from inside and packed the car meticulously, we were on our way to this house somewhere in the mountains. As we drove, I sat in silence and listened to her conversation with her daughter and niece as they played with Barbie dolls in the back. All the way I was thinking of ways I could escape if I needed to. By the time we reached the house and

I was about in a full-blown panic. My heart was beating fiercely, and I was nauseous and sweaty. I then remembered that I had to tell her I could not sleep with anyone in a room.

When we arrived, she put stuff away and chatted with them all and one of the other ladies started cutting her mothers-in-law hair in her kitchen and her other sister-in-law was talking to them as two little blonde girls were playing at her feet. This was going to be a long weekend with a lot of questions. I do not remember much of that weekend other than the fact that I had to tell them I did not sleep well and she said that my roommate had already told her about my sleeping.

Even though there were 4 young girls there they all played extremely well together, and no one screamed at them, or hit them, or hurt them. This was different, could this really be a genuinely good family? It is as if all of them were similar and it would be evident later that the difference was their devotion to the Lord and love for Him and each other that made all the difference. They were genuine followers of Jesus and His Word. This oozed from even their casual conversations. It was unnerving to someone as filled with pain, shame, guilt, fear and terror as myself.

It turned out that I had to sleep on a camp mattress with the sister-in-law and the kids in the same room. So, I did not sleep. I remember staying awake throughout the night and trying to figure out why I was even there.

The next day the kids and I went down to the lower stream that ran behind the house in the woods and looked for crayfish and built stepping bridges across the stream. It was a place that I truly felt comfortable in; the stream in the woods surrounded by the sounds of a deep forest. It reminded me of early days on the hill going with my dad, standing alongside him in the cab as we drove the logging road up to cut wood. These woods and stream were a new sanctuary that in the future would be where a lot of my happy memories would be made, to replace all the terrible ones that had been.

When we returned to the dorm, I was no less quiet or hopeful. It made me feel even more lost and dark to be among those that were spewing forth with goodness, love and this amazing joy. The contrast was palatable. Yes, they were a "good family" to be around. But they certainly were not like me. Nor could I ever see being accepted by them as more than someone to help, a project of sorts.

My roommate was curious at how it went and apologized for throwing me under the bus by ditching me at the last moment. I did not care. I was used to walking alone. Do not rely on others they will always let you down. Fend for yourself and be on guard 24-7. It was safer that way. I told her they had an incredible house and they seemed like a nice family. Too good for me to hang around with.

But God had chosen them. God had chosen me. For such a time as was to come in my life and theirs. It was God, because no one else could orchestrate the events or the hearts that were involved in the coming years. We choose our obedience; He orders our steps.

Much of that year was spent getting to know this family as they attended the college volleyball games, basketball games, softball games and cheered us all on. The lady who worked at the college even joined in our physical education classes when we were playing soccer or racquetball. At times we would come back from an away game and there would be a message on the chalk board in our room. Like "Great game!" or "Don't forget to do your chapel devotions!" This was a strange place. These adults were like none I had ever interacted with before, on so many levels they were caring, free and kind.

My mental state was deteriorating with each passing day without sleep and as much as I tried to catch up with power naps between classes it was not working. The Coach who was also one of my professors of education could tell that I was getting worse. She arranged for yet another free counselor that would by now means understand the gravity or complexity of the abuse I had endured and would not have the tools to help set me free.

They did not know that for me to speak to this novice and it would simply make things worse and not better. My stomach was so sick all the time, I lived on dry bagels or toast and coffee and water. Then it became just dry bagels and water and then nothing but sipping water.

On weekends that I was not being an RA the family asked if I would like to stay with them to get to know them on their turf per se. What their tribe was really like under their own roof and reminded me that her children were not perfect angels. That they would love to host me, and I could leave whenever I liked. They had proven to be kind and after many meetings with the Coach, Dean of Students and the administrator I could sense they really were trying to understand and help.

Why, I was not sure nor am I sure to this day. I was a nobody from a podunk town in the middle of nowhere and had nothing to offer them in return. I could work, that was one thing I was particularly good at. I could clean, mow, garden, paint, shovel, rake, or any other manual labor task they might need. But that was not why they were being kind; they did not want me as their laborer.

The family new I was getting worse so they asked if I would like to join them for thanksgiving break and be their guest at their family thanksgiving. That made me very nervous, because by then I really could not keep a whole lot down or in from all the night terrors and the fear of mother or someone else showing up any moment. I slept on the couch by what I referred to as the campfire, which was really a kerosene heater that just glowed like a campfire.

But I would lay there and stare at it and think about what was going to happen. I would try not to fall asleep as I did not want to have a terror dream a one of their kids would hear and be fearful of me. So, I did all I could stay awake or simply doze and wake myself back up. After that weekend I had to study for finals, and it was hard to function without being able to eat and without sleep. The next weekend I was to stay at their home again as I was off, when I got their I was so weak and tired that I could hardly move once I laid down and they had talked with a family friend who was a psychologist and he said they should take me to the hospital and have me committed to the psych ward for suicidal tendencies. Everything changed.

CHAPTER 9
VOICES OF CONDESCENSION
~ THE PSYCHIATRIC WARD

I was so angry, confused and felt betrayed. I could not understand why they were doing this to me, I was not a mental case. They had no idea. I was just not able to eat. I was not able to keep the food down and my stomach and head always hurt so unbelievably bad!

I had to take this extremely long psych test and answer all these ridiculous questions. There was no way I was going to do their psycho mumbo jumbo and I would do whatever it took to get out of this place and get back to school. The goal was to get a degree, I could not get one in here.

My roommate was getting ready for finals and she said that she could get me if they released me before she headed home for Christmas break. So, I did all the things they asked of me and told them I would be leaving with my roommate at the end of the week. They said that I had to sign a statement that I would have an appointment with a psychologist immediately after my release. I did, my roommate came and picked me up and took me to that family's house, because school was now closed.

Coach came over and sat with them and me and their pastor and his wife and they formed a plan of sorts. I would go to this counselor "friend" of theirs and they would let me stay with them if I did everything he asked. School was closed for break and I had missed finals-I was in no place to bargain. Whatever they asked I would do it. The school let me take in-completes and I was able to retake all the finals over Christmas break and work at the school once again.

The family I was staying with shared they took me there because it was best to get me immediate help and a new direction and they were overwhelmed. When I returned to their house, I was more reserved and did whatever they asked and did my best not to show how I was reeling inside. But at night when I would fall asleep they were then exposed to my night terrors, then mood swings from being sleep deprived and the side effects from the medicine that the hospital put me on and severe stomach pain. I was anxious about them sending me back to the hospital and fearful that those from the valley would take me from school. I spent all break this way and running back and forth to school and work.

Their daughter was always very gracious with her room as they said I should be in a room and not on the couch. She allowed me to sleep on the bottom bunk and never really asked about my night terrors or why I was there-at least not to me. The son was always curious about sports, chess and wanted to hang with his youth group friends most of the time. He accepted me and even at one point was glad I was part of their family life. It was all very foreign, and I was on edge most of the time. Fearful if I messed up that they would kick me out and then I would have no place to live as I no longer was living in the dorms since the hospital stay. They invited me on vacation with them and their extended family that was up at the house in the mountains.

The counselor and his partners, that I was required to see, were once again, not able to deal with the trauma that I shared with them and they switched me to one counselor after the next in their practice until I was with the child psychologist who used small child therapy techniques at a loss of how else to help, and would say "aww that's too bad", and "oh my, how did that make you feel?" Whenever I shared the slightest bit of my story that was the response. It only made things worse and now the family from the valley had gotten word from the school that I was not returning and was committed to the psych ward and now in rehab and staying down to work through these issues. That did not go over well at all! They were furious.

The letters started and then the phone calls, then they came down at one point. That was an awful time. But it showed them that I would not return and that they did not have the power in that area that they had in the valley. They were dealing with authorities and professionals that they could not manipulate or use scare tactics to do whatever they wanted. These therapists were Christian counselors. They had a strength and a protection that was beyond themselves.

CHAPTER 10
VOICES OF CONFUSION
AND MISTRUST

A fter graduating with an associate degree, I went to work for a painter in the area. I could paint and it paid well. I also needed to start paying rent to this family and help more with chores and bills. I then had an experience with one of the supervisors that was off putting and decided I needed to find a different job. I interviewed with a local mortgage company (because I had worked a year in banking to save for college) as a closer. It was the era of the housing market boom and mortgages were closing like wildfire. I was hired on the spot and it was more money than I ever had imagined I would make right out of school. So, I was able to pay them rent, buy groceries, and get some nice dress work clothes so that I looked like the lady that took me in, she always dressed to the nines. I had never seen anyone look like that every day before, and never thought I would have the money to even own one outfit like that, let alone a weeks' worth.

Things were going better with my mind working on numbers all the time, with mandatory overtime and not being at their house much. I was still helping with the youth group now and then, per my associate's degree and still going to the child psychologist per our agreement. Not that she was really helping with the night terrors which continued or with working out the times where I would lose moments, hours or even days in my memory.

That summer I was invited to go with the family I lived with and their extended family at the beach. I had only been twice in my life and both times ended in tragedy, so I was not super excited about going. But, as they talked about what they did at the shore and who all would be there, it sounded different than anything I experienced before.

I asked what I needed to do. I usually did some type of chore or assignment to keep me busy and not having to interact a whole lot with too many people. I just felt like a misfit and that I was nothing like them, I did not belong with this type of people. They were good people, who had loving families, and had this way about them that made me uncomfortable yet drew me in at the same time. There was a part of me that wanted to know them more at the same time wanting to run the other way.

What really made these people live like this? They loved being together all the time with their large extended family. They were always hosting others on Fridays and were always at church. Sunday morning and night, Monday nights, Wednesday Nights. Who does that? They were not getting paid to be there. What was the draw?

It was like a second home to them; they knew everyone, and everyone knew them. They helped missionaries, hosted missionaries, were related to missionaries. They were a family of pastors, teachers, professionals, engineers, and artists. They enjoyed each other. They sang together, went hunting together, worked on their family home in the mountains together, they vacationed together, they lived life together and seemingly never tired of each other.

Even the little cousins felt the same way. They liked each other and never hurt each other or were mean and vicious to each other. They were truly a special family and I was beyond blessed to be a part of that. As uncomfortable as I felt, as different from them as I was, they never made me feel that way. I felt that way because I was different and really like a foreigner in a foreign land.

The only way I can relate the feeling is like a refugee of today. I had come from such severe complex trauma all my life, that being with those that had not been like that nor experienced that nor lived worldly, carnal, lost lives - was like being a hidden refugee in a land of safety.

It is interesting that during this time the lady that initiated me becoming part of this tribe of believers and family introduced me to the Psalms and how David cried out because of the traumas he faced. One night in the middle of the night she came in to get me out of a terror dream and turned to Psalm 90 and 91. That ended up being a chapter that I would read literally hundreds if not a thousand or more times and hold on to the truths in it like a life preserver from that point on to today.

PS 91:1-2 (English Standard Version with my emphasis)
"He (she) who dwells in the shelter of the MOST HIGH will rest in the shadow of the ALMIGHTY. I will say of the LORD, 'He is my refuge, my fortress, my God in whom I trust.'"

CHAPTER 11
VOICES OF FAMILIAR PAIN
~ THE PAST REVISITED

Well, I ended up going with them on that vacation to the shore and one day while the lady and I sat looking out at the waves in silence early one morning, she asked me about writing my father. My biological father. She adored her father and thought maybe if I reached out and at least tried to communicate with him he might be able to explain why he did not rescue me or take me with him. Why was it he fell off the face of the earth like I did not exist? Maybe that would help some of these awful dreams. Maybe he would understand. Maybe he could help. So, I got some paper and wrote a letter asking those things. She found his address somehow and mailed the letter. I never thought he would respond or write or anything. I honestly thought he too had tossed me aside and forgot I was even alive.

But he did respond. He called their house and talked with them. Asked if I was okay and if it would be okay to meet with me. I said I did not want to go back there and felt nauseous about the whole thing. He was not supposed to respond. She set up a place halfway between us to meet and they took me there to meet with him; they had a pastor friend at that halfway point and were planning on spending some time with them as well.

He looked the same as I remembered but older, his wife was

quite different then mother and bubbly and kind. He sat at that restaurant table and smoked his pipe (that smell-brought back a flood of memories-these good) then he started flipping and tapping his stainless-steel lighter on the table. I remember that! I remember whenever he would be sitting at a table, he did that. The lady chatted with him for quite some time and I talked a little about where I had gone to school and my job. Then we parted ways and he said he hoped to see me again sometime. He gave me a hug, I was not much of a hugger, I hated to be held like that, I detested being touched. He smelled exactly like I remember, pipe smoke, old spice, wood and motor grease. I thought that was the last time I would see him again and it was fine. But as it turned out there would be another time.

That moment would come sooner than I had thought. Because after a long fall and new attempts the following spring from grandmother and mother and my half-brother to convince us that they had changed and that since mother's brain aneurysm she was a different person and now wanted me to come back to show me that she could be different; I caved.

On top of that the counselor that I was seeing then, had already began convincing me it was my place to go back and save them. If others up there just knew the truth and the Good News of the Gospel- they certainly would be set free too.

GOOD FOR WHOM?

Somehow, we all believed that or somewhere in all those involved they wanted to believe that was true. The warlock had been gone now for several months; arrested and taken back to where he came from. Mother had quickly remarried an older widower. This man was wealthy for that area and had an apartment in the upstairs of his house that I could rent cheap and get back to where I came from and belonged. When I got there, they repeatedly reminded me to remember this fact of who I was and that this is where I belonged. It would become a prison once again.

That was a double hit for my brain, I was told to go back and fight and save them for Christ and now they were here saying they had changed and that I did not belong here but there. I am not sure how they fooled the people I was living with, just out of sheer exhaustion with my situation and me as a whole or if they truly believed this was best. Either way, I gave my two weeks' notice at the mortgage company and set off the fight the battle against the enemy with no real weapons of my own and just some ridiculous notion that I could make them see how this way of life was evil and would lead to eternal hell. That you should not play with witchcraft and the occult and that they can have a better life. I see now how foolish this all was. I had nothing within myself at that point to fight this very real battle and I would only suffer more mental and emotional wounds from this choice that I made and regret on many levels.

The new counselor referred by the one that could no longer handle the gravity of my case was a former pastor turned ritualistic abuse counselor, and he said that it was my duty as a Christian and as a child to work things out with them now that I was an adult and that I should go up and fight the enemy and win them to the Lord. That I would be a coward and a failure if I ran away from this battle. This was no one else's battle but mine and I could not expect any of the dreams or trauma to be healed until I dealt with the source of it. I had to cut the head of the source of my trauma off and it was the hold of the enemy in that area that was the source.

Not the best advice. I was already prone to want to defend them and be their savior, and would truly suffer for listening to him, believing he was a pastor as well as a counselor and certainly knew better than I did what the Lord would want me to do. I did not want to shrink back and I had always had an extreme sense of duty to mother and guilt for "dishonoring" her by even speaking of the sexual abuse and ritualistic abuse that I suffered at her hands and those of the ones she gave me to.

I also did not want to be a burden and have the Lord be ashamed of me when He returned. I would pack the meager belongings I had and would head to the valley. I would start a ministry that would help youth who were going through the same things. I had been convinced that only I could do this-only I could fight the enemy- he wanted me-not these people to wage this war and win. If I went the Valley could be changed and God would have their hearts and we would all be free and reconciled in every way. This is what I told myself as I prepared to go and leave the safety of this new family. These were lies that I believed and walked in, into a fiery trap. If I had stopped and really prayed about it, maybe I would have seen more clearly. But I was not in a place to do that. I was not free, I was not healed, I was simply wearing one of many masks that I was a master of more than I even knew. What was I or that counselor thinking?! How could I possible show the way to freedom or healing for others-I could not, and it would only make my trauma worse.

ALONE IN ENEMY TERRITORY AND UNWELL

But, just as the car issue brought about good things so did this time of return to the enemy's ground. I saw firsthand that things had not changed, and that I was not the one to bring the gospel. I was not well received by the "church" there nor did they want anything to do with a ministry to those who had been abused. They would not listen to my story and they would not confront either mother or the others, I was not to say that I had been abused. This was hopeless, the elders that I spoke with were truly angry with me and wondered how could I tell those people about our life in the valley?

Those people knew nothing of this place and how things

worked. I just better get down off my high horse and accept who I am, where I came from and now that I returned - that I will always be in this valley and do what I am told. I felt hopeless and trapped after that meeting. I was not accepted as one to bring healing and hope to those who were living there.

Even though there was one other adult who, from an adjoining town, who had thought it was a great idea-no one else did. The youth leaders from the forbidden church I had attended at the end of high school did not receive me back with open arms either. They actually looked at me and asked "What are YOU doing back here?! We did not want you to come back here!" I felt alone and a failure and lost in darkness once again,

The blessing is this: I did get to see my father and his new bubbly wife again and understand a little more about all that he had been through and that he too was getting out and moving away as soon as he was able. He did just that and to the area she was from and as far as I know they got exactly what they wanted. I never saw him again after that time as I would not become part of the secret society that he was part of and wanted all his natural kids to be part of to pass down the secrets and the books that were part of it. He gave me a book that looked like a bible of sorts, which had my name in the long list of ancestors.

I loved my Dad very much and I thought it was kind of him to give it to me. I took it and hid it in a box of keepsakes that I would take when I got out again. I said I was a Christian and that I wanted no part of that. He said he was too, and that I did not understand the importance of being a part of this society. It was powerful, important and basically followed the Bible. I said I would not become a part of the woman's division and that I wanted to help others and go back to Bible College. He gave up and said fine and when I left that evening it was clear that he did not want to have anything to do with me from then on. I regret never reconciling with him before he died. I was so broken and lost, and desperate to just get free from the hold of that place once again.

I decided the only way back out was like before, schooling. I started putting out applications to different Christian schools that would be affordable for me or had a work study program and who could take the credits from my associates so I would not need to start over.

In the middle of doing this and working at the job that I had gotten which was within walking distance of the place I was living with mother and her new husband. The job was perfect because it was in a back office doing accounting and payrolls. I was very thankful that I had worked in the bank for a year before saving enough to go to school the first time, and the mortgage company. I have learned that each experience the Lord allows in our lives can be built on at another point. I worked mostly by myself as the guys were out in the field planting trees and putting together timber management plans. Which was remarkably interesting to me, I do love to learn. I learned how to calculate board feet from the diameter and height of the straight timber of a tree. Interesting to my every curious mind.

Then one summer night right before Memorial Day weekend, my appendix ruptured, and I was sick throwing up for a whole week because the small-town doctor thought it was just the flu. At the end of the week he sent me to the nearest hospital that was a good distance away. They confirmed the appendix had ruptured the night I sat up in severe pain and started throwing up and that now part of my colon on either side was completely gangrene and would need to be removed. I was in the hospital for a couple of weeks. Resting and thinking how long I would be in this place in this valley and why did I ever come back. I should have never listened to that guy or my own undiscerning brain! This is what I deserve.

Recovery was interesting in a house where you are being endured, mother's prior nature before I left was coming out more and more. Her dog was frightening and would try to attack me often, and almost got me one day. It was a big mean breed known for being vicious and it was, how fitting. Because of my finances and who I was, I could not find a way to live somewhere else and pay for school. Their attic apartment would have to do.

I had survived worse and the new guy was not threatening at all. He was oblivious in so many ways and mother's 5th husband at this point, he was a much older man with a calm demeanor. He would usually just sit watch fights and drink and do whatever mother wanted. So, unlike the warlock and the other men she had my entire growing up. But this man was also very wealthy for that area and she was getting older and no longer able to draw men in to take care of her, nor could she work any longer as she was now on disability from a fall down a stairwell at her former place of employment which revealed that she had brain a brain aneurysm. Honestly, I am not sure he even knew all her story or her past or even our history at all, other than who her mother was, and that she was extremely intelligent. Or he did, and he simply did not care nor need to.

By the end of that summer I had secured several college acceptances to fall programs. I was so thankful that I would continue schooling and get another degree that would secure my hopes of being free of all this torment for good! And this time I would never return, I would not be fooled again into believing a lie of changes that were made by others or that I could make them see truth and want to change a whole people group that had lived in these patterns for generations. It was not for me to do. The Lord certainly could, and I do pray that He has destroyed all the works of the enemy in that area and set those families free.

It seemed like once I had arrived there, I lost all levels of confidence, as well as any hope I had mustered that I could ever begin to make a change in the community or even any other youth's life.

I would have terrible debilitating headaches. To escape the oppression in the house I would spend a lot of time riding my bike and trying to formulate a plan to get out once again. I was by no means the one to bring hope and healing to this valley. No, I was as always simply the pawn of mother and her directions or grandmother and her manipulation. I could not go against them; I would go mute whenever I tried to rebut what they said or speak against their lifestyle or address the past and the abuse. I was powerless against their presence. I was not free at that point and had not completely surrendered to the Lord and His authority in my life.

I would just withdraw within and wait out my time. The Warlock, I was told, had been arrested and was no longer in the area for at least the next 10-20 years. I was still very vulnerable, and mother used this sense of fear, duty and guilt as a leverage in mind games and verbal abuse.

That counselor was quite off base and it only served to be a time of more suffering and confusion and an inroad for more darkness to grab hold of my brain and hopelessness to grow in my heart. Both were enough to begin to smother the little flicker, of the light of truth, that had begun to spark in my heart before coming back to this place.

One day, while I was there recovering from my appendectomy and bowel restructuring in that attic apartment, I began trying to get an old form of a desktop computer to work, I broke down in frustration! I stopped and sat on my bed with my head in my hands overwhelmed with even being there again and like everything else, my failure and this old computer was the last mental straw. I was anxious to the core not knowing when I would be able to leave and simply sat there and cried and began to pray and ask the Lord what was next and what I was to do??

At that moment in my gut, and as if someone physically whispered to me, a name came clearly in my mind. Very random and intense was this incident and the impression was that it was the name of the person I would marry.

What?! No way!! One, I am never ever getting married! Two, the only guy I knew with that name was a drug dealer and he was usually mentally incapacitated most the time. But, like most things in my life, it was not for that immediate time. To my shock and amazement, just three years later I would indeed meet someone else with that name, quite far from this valley, and in an additional three years later would marry him. Only God! His sovereignty and power know no bounds!

THIS WORD HE SPOKE AND IS TRUE AND REMAINS FOREVER!

Jeremiah 29:8-11, 13-14 (New Living Translation)
"This is what the Lord of Heaven's Armies, the God of Israel, says: "Do not let your prophets and fortune-tellers who are with you in the land of Babylon trick you. Do not listen to their dreams, because they are telling you lies in my name. I have not sent them," says the Lord. This is what the Lord says: "You will be in Babylon for seventy years. But then I will come and do for you all the good things I have promised, and I will bring you home again. For I know the plans I have for you," says the Lord. "They are plans for good and not for disaster, to give you a future and a hope. If you look for me wholeheartedly, you will find me. I will be found by you," says the Lord. "I will end your captivity and restore your fortunes. I will gather you out of the nations where I sent you and will bring you home again to your own land.""

He did and He does! He has a plan; He can be found when you seek after Him and He alone safely brings us out of captivity...even a captivity we ourselves have created by choosing to believe a lie or by repeatedly deceiving ourselves. For He is Jehovah Sabaoth - The LORD of Heaven's Armies! He alone can completely rewrite our future if we will only let Him!

CHAPTER 12
VOICES OF FALSE HOPE
~ POOR DECISIONS

The one school that I did want to go to was far away on the other side of the country, and would not accept my credits nor were they themselves accredited. I was so disheartened, but I knew that not getting a valid education would not serve me well. I chose the one back in the area where I had gone before, hoping that it would be safe and as good as before and that this time I would make the most of the opportunity and keep to myself focused on success and just work and study.

I was good at that. I was a task-oriented introvert, so this plan seemed good to me at the time and I did not want to hurt or bother anyone else. If I was alone than no one would be bothered by my night terrors and no one would ask me questions and I could just push through this life.

By now I figured that the family that I had lived with before really did not want or could not handle me anymore and that they had had enough. They had given a couple of years of their lives to help me and now I must fight through the rest of this life on my own again. I have made some extremely foolish decisions in my self-sufficient, prideful protectiveness. I was about to make another one.

I had accepted an offer to live with a lady that had originally been from the valley but was relocated now some 15 years at least to that area. She said she was a Christian now and just wanted to help me out and give me a chance at a different life too. She was athletic and some others from the church that I went to when I was going to school before knew her and thought it should be a good match. We would "get" each other's odd quirks. Well, I started a full-time job as a secretary and went to college full-time too, I would not be around much so this would work. It only took a little over a month before things went very south.

I should have been wiser and steered clear of anyone or anything that had ever been associated with the valley. Especially, currently so soon after getting out once again. She wanted to have a "relationship" with me that required me to always check with her whenever I was leaving school and let her know who I talked to that day and what I told them. She then began forbidding me to stay at school to study or to see other people from school on the weekends. I was to spend any off time with her.

One night after studying for an exam and working on the paper in the school library until it closed 11pm ~I drove back and she was standing there, waiting in the driveway. She ripped open my door and very angrily asked where I had been, then she said I was not leaving the house again. I panicked out! I tried to close the door, but she held on to it, I had not taken off my seatbelt and just slammed the car in reverse and started backing away fast! She had to let go! She screamed something as I drove away. I really had no idea where I was going to go, just drive!

I ended up back at the church, it seemed the safest place to go. So that night I slept in my car in the church parking lot not knowing what to do next. It was the weekend so I would need to find a place to stay. How was I going to get my clothes and other books from her house? She certainly will not just "give" them to me.

I called my former Coach who also still lived in the area and asked for help. She was strong and scared me so I figured she would be the perfect one to help me if she would. I explained what happened as best I could, and she agreed it was weird and I should not stay there any longer. She did more than help me get my things back...she offered to let me stay with them for the rest of that school year. She also was my former professor, so she was aware of my drive to study and excel. They extended the hospitality of their home and a room they called the Elijah room. Very fitting indeed for this couple. God was continuing to show me His provision and care- even in my stubbornness, hiding and aloneness.

The full-time secretary job began getting very scary. The president that I worked for would ask us to do some unethical things with the bid packages and he would call me into his office to scream at me. Then I found out that he had purchased 600 acres in of all places the valley, from a farmer's family that had died and he had hired my half-brother to clear the roads for him. WHAT?!!!! How is this even possible? What were the chances? How would he even know about this area, let alone be hiring unbeknownst to him my half-brother?

Again, I knew that I was being watched and that I was not free even though I was hundreds of miles away. I knew that I needed to resign and yet did not want to make it known why. I found another position as a back-office administrator of finances for a doctor's office where my apartment was to be. I resigned and began training for the new position as well as finishing what would be my last semester of school.

School was going very well and I was getting great grades and loving the Bible and education classes. This new college was much bigger than the one where I had attended previously and received my associates; it had so many more classes and the library was amazing. I would stay after class until it closed, working there instead of the commuter lounge, to get my work done. It was the perfect setting as it was quiet, all the resources were right there, and no one would talk to me.

My focus was on getting good grades and learning not on making friends or talking with anyone. I finished that year with a 4.0 and was excited. Then I got the financial aid transcript of the estimated costs of the next and final year and I was devastated. There was no way I could pay that! I could not possibly work anymore and there was no way I was going into more debt. I already had $13,000 plus dollars waiting for me to pay off from this whole year and the remainder of my first school. I could not continue. But at least I could work and work at the church as a youth leader. I guess that is all I was to be. I was disheartened about not being able to go back. Just because of money.

It was for the best as I look back now. The dreams were getting worse and there were nights I had no recollection of driving home from class. There were days I completely missed or did not remember. I was getting worse and trying desperately not to let anyone know. Without classes to focus on and time in a library I was not sure how I would do. Working more at the church when others were there would mean that I would be around people and that was extremely uncomfortable.

By the end of that semester it was clear that I really needed to be in my own apartment. The couple wanted to start a family, and I was getting edgy being there especially when they would have other people over or their family over. They were a very busy, hospitable, generous couple and being around different people, all the time made me feel even more uneasy and anxious so I would tend to stay in the room or go for a walk or bike ride when other people were there and became increasingly more withdrawn.

I found an efficiency apartment in town, and by now was working as an assistant to the youth pastor at the church as well as my new position at the doctor's office. This apartment was located under a very busy bar/restaurant and I would find out that the I was paying for the electric for their freezers and half of their equipment. The electrical cost was outrageous for an efficiency apartment! Then I had an idea to try to figure out why this could be and one day when I went to work, I simply shut the breaker off - I had nothing in my refrigerator so there was nothing to spoil.

When I came back from work, all these guys were in the other side large room cursing and yelling about all their freezers thawing. That confirmed it. They had tapped into my electric. So, I called the landlord and he had the electric company come out and change the boxes and put theirs on their wall. I felt like after that they were disgruntled and I was super uneasy pulling in from work late, because I never knew who could be in the parking lot waiting. Another added stress to my already anxious mind.

CHAPTER 13
VOICES FROM WITHIN
~ NIGHT TERRORS AND
FLASHBACKS

The frequency of flashbacks and terror dreams increased in the apartment and I would lose days at a time when I would not remember how I got where I was or what I did. I longed to be at church, it was a place I felt like these things could not reach me or have power over me there. So I would go very early on Sundays to the youth office at the church to put together the youth bulletins and work on our meeting schedules and any other odds and ends that needed to be done. Just to keep focused and busy in the church. I felt the safest there, that church was a sanctuary for me.

The body there was large by my standards, but not by the area's standards. It was easy enough to get lost in just doing things. The youth pastor and his new wife were not only my supervisors but friends as well by then. They were kind, funny, very outdoorsy and enjoyed teaching the youth. You could see they really wanted the best for these kids, they had a real passion to teach them the Bible and how to apply it to their lives. This was something I was thankful to be a little part of and personally had never experienced.

"Peculiar" is the word the older members of that congregation used to describe me. Or that girl over there that so and so use to let live with them. They were not shy about it either. It is as if when you reached a certain age, unkind words were okay for you to say to others, simply because you were elderly.

It still stung like a wasp and I can still hear their tones in their voices today although all those people have now died. This type of talk is yet another level of cutting voices that are used to destroy and not build up. They certainly had not chosen to edify the young and hurting, but to judge and segregate instead. Those words and memory of their voices would haunt me whenever I walked in that hallway and even when I would much later in life visit that church, this is one of the things I think of as I enter the old hallways.

TALK TO SOMEONE PLEASE

One Sunday one of the pastors of the church came in early to pray over the pews and the building. He had made a practice of praying like this on Sunday mornings. His voice was very calming and yet authoritative. I was both intrigued and frightened if that makes sense. He was a particularly good friend of the family that had taken me in those first years of beginning transformation. So, I was not fearful of him as I had already had plenty of interaction outside the church with them and he and his family, prior to this interaction.

He leaned in the doorway and asked what I was doing here so early-again. I told him I was working on the bulletins for the youth so they would be ready when they came. Did he have any changes that he or the head pastor needed me to include? I remember that conversation like it was yesterday. I can even see the office and the long tank where the youth pastor kept his - uhm pets...I did not particular care for that tank. He then said that he thought that I needed to "talk to somebody". I said I was fine and that if I worked and focused on school, youth and work I could keep going. He said well if you will not talk with me, I would like you to talk to someone who could help you. I looked like I could use some much-needed sleep and find out what was causing me such turmoil. I said I would think about it.

He left and a little while later he came back down and put two brochures on the desk in front of me and said to at least call one of these people. Well, the one was a man and seemed expensive and the other was a woman and was far away. I did not think either would work. But, I did not want to lose my job with the youth by being out of it when we were supposed to be examples and teachers, and I loved just simply being in the church itself when no one else was there.

So, I went back to my apartment and put the brochures on the counter and paced. Paced and thought how dangerous and thoughtless it would be for me to try to talk to anyone again. I am sure he meant well, but he had no idea what they could do, or might do if I ever told my story. That is often what I did for a good part of the time that I was inside that place. Pace, and think and worry and then, I would get on my bike and ride and ride and ride. Thinking and thinking and trying to figure out how I could fix myself and what to do next. I went back to the brochures and looked at them. They would have to wait. I could not talk to anyone now, not even on the phone. I was too keyed up.

I went for a drive and ended up at the lake where, often, it would feel like it was calling me into it. I sat by the pier and looked out over it and just got lost in the mesmerizing black-green ripples of water, staring and thinking what to do, what to do. It was getting dark and the park was closed but I could still drive out. I had not produced an alternative plan. I had no idea how to make the images and the endless terror dreams and flashbacks stop - I had tried repeatedly. Nothing had worked for me.

I left and came back to the apartment- the brochures were

still there. I would deal with them tomorrow before I saw the other pastor, who was sure to ask if I had called or even looked at them. I am by nature a peace keeper and never want to upset anyone, this was my bent for was as far back as I could remember and now was no different than when I was small. I had learned early to obey immediately or the consequences were painful. That trait has served both as a blessing and a curse. I tend to have a good relationship with most people, but at the cost of self often.

When I went to lay down on the couch, I could hear his voice saying, "You need to talk to somebody." It kept replaying in my brain and then, as if out of the walls there were these awful voices reminding me if I did, if I ever said anything to these people I would die. They will kill me, I was cursed. At a noticeably young age, they had convinced me that they knew everything I said and who I said it to, and they watched my every move.

I began shaking again like many nights before and would "see" the warlock in the room and relive the trauma of my childhood over again. The knife coming through the door, his cold hands and his evil voice and the alcohol/drug laden breath and smell. I would scream and no one would come. I would scream and no one would come. I would scream and no one would come and no one every would. That is what I learned. I did not believe I would ever be free from them or safe or at peace.

I was up all night with those kinds of voices and terror dreams and flashbacks. When I went into work at the office the next day the doctor and the office manager both said I looked extremely sick and should I go home and rest. I said, "NO!" I knew it would not get any better there at the apartment.

They were both believers and understood more what I was going through than I knew at the time. The family I had lived with in college as well as the couple I had stayed with during the college year had informed them of some of my struggles and they were very gracious and kind to me as both employers as well as fellow believers.

CHAPTER 14

THE VOICE THAT WHISPERS ~ FREEDOM AND THE TRUTH

When I went home after work the brochures were in the same place. So, I called the one on top, and he was not available it went to voicemail and I hung up. He was a man and there was nothing in me that wanted to sit in any office alone with a door shut with a man or a strange woman for that matter. Well, I had to go to the church to work so I better call this other number. It was fairly far away though. I called and the receptionist picked up right away. I swallowed. Her voice seemed soft and controlled. Not weird or anything, just sweet you might say.

I told her that the church where I was working gave me the therapists brochure and told me I was should talk to her. She apologized and said that she was sorry, she was not accepting any new patients. (Whew!) Well, I had done what I was asked, and it was just not meant to be I thought...

The receptionist then asked if she could take my name and what I wanted help with to see if one of the other therapists would be available. I said, no thank you that it was okay. She again asked for my name, so I gave her my name (I still am not sure why) and she asked me to hold. At that point I was ready to just hang up. She would never be able to reach me. This was an age before caller ID or cell phones. I hung up the receiver on the telephone that hung on the wall attached by a cord. Back in the old days as you might say. But I did not hang up and she came back on the line and said could I please wait a moment that the doctor was in a conference call about me and did indeed want to schedule an appointment.

I asked how she even knew about me let alone be on another phone call with someone about me. Then I started to get really suspicious and frightened remembering what the voices the night before had said. Could this all be a trick? Maybe it was someone from the valley? No none of those things were accurate; the receptionist said the name and it was actually the pastor that had given me the brochure and someone else, whom to this day I cannot remember who she said it was. Well, now I was stuck. I did what I was asked and now I was also going to need to follow-through. The receptionists set up the initial intake appointment and the rest is, as you say, history. If it were only that quick and easy. But nothing worth gaining is done quickly - and I desperately wanted these night terrors and flashbacks to stop-so I would start at least.

This was the best decision that I made and the Lord had clearly led and prepared the way for the doctor, the pastor and prayer team to travel faithfully toward healing with me and all the long years of battling for my life that lay ahead.

DR. PAIN AND PRICELESS IN THE END

At first, I nicknamed her "doctor pain", she transitioned through the years of intense therapy and intense fervent prayer and work to be called "doctor priceless" and a tool of Our Lord Jehovah Raphe. The God Who heals. She was a blessing and a tool of the Master Physician and I am eternally grateful He orchestrated that appointment. Indeed, the enemy has no power on earth that can thwart His redemptive plan. Praise Jesus His is Victor!! His work on the cross on our behalf changes everything! There is no valley too deep, too dark, too long, too crooked, too old that He cannot and will not either lead you through to the other side or carry you through or both!!

Honestly, there is so much that happened in the next years that this chapter will be absolutely full of so many new voices from a plethora of new people and places.

The next few years will be a time of extreme pain, with the blessing of limitless gain and setting free, and metamorphosis of self that the Creator of the Universe had ordained before the world began. There is no way to fully wrap my mind around what has happened in and to me, or even in and through me. But GOD. Is indescribable and immutable. His Word is indeed living and active and powerful to set the captives free and His truth demolishes strongholds and years of captivity to lies and fear.

The One Who set me free was Jesus Christ the Son of the Living God - and when the Son sets you free, you are free indeed! It is the living out of that freedom and the acceptance of an undeserved but wonderfully gracious new identity that takes years.

In fact, we continue to change from glory to glory, freedom to freedom like peeling an onion-until He returns for us or takes us home. Then we will be like Him and we will be completely transformed in a twinkling of an eye into who He created us to be in all His glory! Falling at His feet in worship and awe and adoration for all my days!

The war is won by many vicious, yet in the end, victorious battles...and the first one that was to be the beginning of the end of captivity was the first initial intake session. This session was a battle just to get to physically, mentally, emotionally and spiritually.

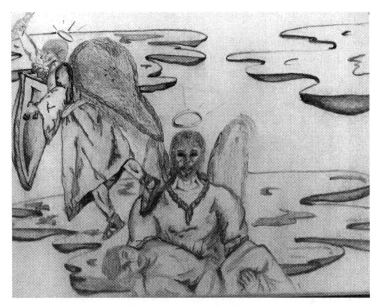

Figure 5- His Angelic Holy Army battles for you!

Physically, I did not know where I was going, and it was driving into a city which I was not comfortable with at all. Mentally was figuring our why I needed to be doing this and that battle raged within and was a thousand times harder than the traffic I was faced with. Spiritually, were the past voices that loved darkness and hiding and twisted threats, those that spewed curses and screamed and wanted me to turn around, reminding me they would kill me if I opened my mouth. Emotionally, I was numb to others and the outside, I worked extremely hard at not feeling.

Logically my brain was remembering the past failures in the counseling realm on my behalf. Then an overwhelming wave of dread that this person was no different than any of the other counselors, psychiatrists or therapists. That this one like the others, would just make things worse and she probably could not handle the things that were really going on in my head and heart and past. Battle one of numberless others to come, be waged and won before the real victory was won and this war over!

But, as with any battle - the first line of attack is knowing who the enemy is- it is this unknown and determining who they are and their weaknesses, that can either give your insight that leads to victory or false information that leads to deeper captivity and loss.

Gratefully, looking back at it all, the Lord was in charge. Jesus was the One making it clear that my enemy was not the counselor, nor the receptionist, pastor, sponsor or even the abusers. The real enemy was Satan, the enemy of our souls. Jesus had secured my true victory long ago, I just had not fully grasped all that meant.

Only Jesus could open my eyes to see this and my heart to accept His fighting for me and His victory. I would need to do some hard work to reverse the damage of real people and a life of complex trauma. But He would be my strength and lifter of my head through each and every battle. It was all Him whether I was aware of it at the time or not. What He promises in His Word He fulfills. This I now know to be absolutely true!

I made it to her office and sat in the parking lot raging within. It would take more than I could muster to walk in that office. But the next thing I remember is filling out paperwork and sitting in this small foyer that looked like a room out of an 1800's colonial documentary. This would be too expensive. There is no way I can do this. What am I doing here? The next thing I remember, was that I was sitting on a couch, it was a lovely couch that fit the era of the home the office was located in. I counted the flowers on the cover and then the dots on the pillow, I saw her lips moving but could not really hear what she was saying. I was not talking, there was no way to talk. If I did, they would kill me and her. That is what the voices, which I could hear loud and clear, kept repeating over and over in my head in tones that just oozed evil.

I left and the next thing I knew I was in my apartment screaming for the image before me to leave me alone, to please stop hitting me, I was sorry please stop, stop hurting me. I said I had not said anything and that I was just there and that I had to go. Then I woke up and it was time for work again. This would be the way it would go for the next several appointments. Me making it there, not being able to speak, and leaving and going through terrible flashbacks, panic attacks and terror dreams.

THE BIG CHOICE OF A SPONSOR

Finally, one session shortly after we began, she said that I needed to have a sponsor. Someone to walk with me through this process. Did I know anyone I trusted or was willing to take on this type of a role? Willing to bring me to the appointments and monitor me during the times we were not meeting. Also, she had made a tape of her voice, steps to focus on reality of things in a room and scripture to help me get use to the safety of it and the power to escape from flashbacks or terror dream effects. I still have that cassette. It is a war medal of sorts.

By this time, I had been involved in the family that had taken me in during college for some family functions and I knew the head pastor's wife and of course the youth pastor's wife. There were certain strengths in all of them and I had seen how they handled their kids, and the struggles with those from the valley who had been involved in my life. So, I chose two, amongst all of them, to ask.

There was a lady at the place where I worked that heard from the doctor, I worked for that I needed a sponsor. She asked if she could be that, and I said emphatically, NO! She had already become so controlling and micromanaging at work, I could not imagine that in hours outside of work. I was struggling to ask the other two because I simply hated, hated, hated to ask for help in any way. Plus, I knew that this would mean they would be in danger themselves. I would just tell them that, and then let the chips fall where they may. Certainly, they would not want to take this on once they knew the danger, they would be in.

I asked the pastor's wife first on a walk at lunchtime. She would often ask me to walk with her and the secretary, who was the lady of the family that took me in during the first years at college. I was grateful to be included in the walks though, because I hated being inside. The one thing that really stood out to me was that they always prayed for me and encouraged me to be reading my bible and praying as well.

Neither of those things that they suggested were easy for me to do on my own. Because when I would open up the Bible, that the lady from my first college years, gave me for my 21st birthday (with my nickname engraved on the front cover and in my favorite color and pattern one of the most thoughtful and nicest gifts I had received up to that point in my life) I would here a cacophony of voices (some were simply mother's and grandmother's asking if I thought I was better than they were and others were unnerving creepy screams and cursing) that made it difficult to read and pray by myself. There was no way I would tell them that though, I did not want to every go back to a psyche unit and be treated the way I was treated in college. I was not mentally ill- I had a raging battle within and it would take one mega ton J-bomb to squelch the enemy that led the troops against me in my mind and heart, they were fierce and always in my dreams.

One Wednesday when I had off work (lots of doctors' offices in this area were closed on Wednesdays- I have no idea why) I stopped by the church and only she was there. Perfect. I asked if she wanted to go for a quick walk. Oh, sure she said. We walked down the lane and she chatted about what was going on in the church, her family and preschool and I walked quietly, just listening and taking it all in. I thought this was not the time to ask.

She had so much she was already carrying and although her personality and trustworthiness were perfect, she already had enough. She asked if I was continuing with the counselor that the other pastor had suggested? I said that I was and was needing to ask her a question and that I already thought she had enough going on in her life, but I needed to find a sponsor to start the next part of therapy according to the doctor. She said that she would absolutely pray for me through it and had been. They had asked several trustworthy people to pray in fact. They knew this was going to be difficult.

So, the only other one that I thought had the strength, consistent personality grounded spiritually, and a heritage of godliness was asked. I asked her on a walk as well. This memory was lost to me and I had to ask her how I asked her. There is so much of this time that I do not remember with clarity. Especially when it involves points of transition or battles. I remember up to the time, then the after time, but the battle itself and the setting free is lost. I think that may be a gift. Because my memory of times, people and events goes back to about 3 years old. But these recent memories of crucial things and spiritual battles - the details are lost on some of them. Others are very vivid!

She agreed and the work began in me immediately, the task of just trusting her enough to allow her to go with me to the appointments was overwhelming at first and I would get all angry and guarded. Responding out of fear and insecurity.

This was not helpful and I would need to trust her. But, why did I need yet another person? Why could I not fight this on my own by my own strength? I thought that I was fairly strong physically. I biked a lot and lifted weights. I played sports year-round and I was highly competitive. I played to win. This could be like a racquetball match, I just needed to figure out the best angle and get the kill shot.

But, honestly, it turned out to be a long distance spartan race with no end in sight. There was no way I was in any way truly prepared for the battles or the length of time nor the enemy that I had to face.

This was one of those times where it is best that we do not know what lies ahead.

VOICE OF THE REDEEMER
~ HIS WORD AND HIS PEOPLE

Work done in that office over the course of the next several years is without question the hardest and longest toiling I have ever done on this earth or will ever do. In all honestly it was not in my strength that any of it was carried out. Every moment, the whole of it was accomplished by the hand of the Lord Jesus, His Word and His servant's obedience and faithful prayers lifted and directed to the Throne of Mercy through the indwelling Mighty Holy Spirit on my behalf.

For these things I am eternally, truly, eternally grateful. For because of His Faithfulness and Great Grace, the power of His shed blood, and the testimony of the truth of the gospel. I, a shattered piece of darkly stained glass, have been carefully and completely cleansed, reshaped and made whole. Why? So that He can shine through me to bring hope and the truth of His redemption to others. For He wishes that none perish. But that all come to salvation and eternal life through His Son the Lord Jesus!

The arduous trek toward healing and wholeness is difficult to type. Just as it was years of terrifying trauma, so it would be years of difficult work to reveal and heal.

Doctor Pain would see me two to three times a week and the pastor who had dropped the brochure on the desk that Sunday morning would also see me one to two times a week. The sponsor would check on me routinely.

I had come to such a point of not being able to function that the youth pastor and his wife moved me in with them at their large apartment in a more rural setting. Then they moved into the adjoining larger town when they bought their first home. It was helpful financially to board with them, and they were part of the key prayer team that was formed. But, the dreams and flashbacks, my own uneasiness at living with yet another couple was weighing heavy and the sponsor could not adequately check my progress or regress. So, in time I was offered to stay with the sponsor and her family.

To say that by now I had truly little belongings is an understatement. I only had a few boxes of books and my clothes. There were items from the apartment that were given to me a couch, 1950s dinette table with 2 chairs, a small heater. I had my bike and when I moved in with them that is what I missed most. The sponsor lived even more rural than the youth pastor's apartment. There was no way that I felt comfortable riding my bike out there, there were too many cars and no shoulder on the roads.

THE BODY OF CHRIST WORKING PROPERLY

The church that I was working with the youth at and had been attending, formed a prayer team to cover me and all those involved in my healing process through this time. This is an amazing visual portrayal of the working of the Body of Christ on behalf of a weaker sister to bring her to healing and wholeness. They were, and still are, each priceless in my heart and life. That's been a lifetime ago it seems, and many of us are no longer worshipping in the same building together ~ but we are eternally brothers and sisters, children of The Most High God and of One Body, of which Christ Jesus is the Head.

Prayer was and is an amazingly personal and mighty weapon

for the Lord's people throughout His story. I would come to find out how immensely powerful and intimate that this tool is from God the Father to His children. He calls us to seek Him, with all our hearts and minds; and when we truly do seek Him, He may be found! King David exhorted the wisest man to ever live, his son Solomon with this same truth:

I CHRONICLES 16:11 (NIV)
"Look to the Lord and His strength; seek His face always."

I CHRONICLES 28:9 (NIV)
"And you, my son Solomon, acknowledge the God of your father, and serve Him with wholehearted devotion and with a willing mind, for the Lord searches the heart and understands every motive behind the thoughts. IF YOU SEEK HIM, HE WILL BE FOUND BY YOU."

Jesus made it clear that we are to pray and never give up.

LUKE 18:1 (NIV)
"Then Jesus told His disciples a parable to show them that they should always pray and never give up."

This never giving up amid unbelievable pain and sorrow is something He was the King of! He not only prayed to the Father while He was preparing for the biggest battle of all time in the Garden at Gethsemane- He would often go our alone early in the morning to pray while He walked here with us. By His great grace and gift, through the strength of His Spirit, we are able to do the same.

In the midst of intense therapy session and the after work that I had to do (journaling, drawing, speaking truth out loud, listening to the scripture tapes and truth tapes) there were many times I wanted to be done, to give up, to just curl up in a ball and go to sleep and never wake up. To go to the lake and just walk in and keep walking until I was no longer here.

It seemed so very many times that this was all too hard to face again and again until it was conquered. Without the prayers of His people and my seeking Him out of fear and desperation and the intercession of the Holy Spirit and He Himself ultimately-I would have never had the strength to push through the battles and emerge with Him safely on the other side of healing.

Graciously, God gave me His very gifted and wise children to walk with me this time in the present reality. He shone His light on the darkness of the repeated abuse. Looking at the trauma with the eyes of an adult filled me with a powerful sense of loss and unbelievable anger. I had been numb to emotions and to even healthy feeling for a reason. This was it. This seemed way too hard to carry and to conquer. BUT GOD~HE HAS THE FINAL SAY! The process of carrying it to His feet is what finally healed me and made me whole and of sound mind again.

> *EPHESIANS 4:16* (ESV)
> "From HIM the whole body, joined together by
> every supporting ligament, grows and builds itself
> up in love, as each part does its work"

IT TAKES A TEAM AND A LONGTERM COMMITTMENT

Those involved in this intense time of revealing and healing were directed by The Redeemer and each of them certainly did their work. It was by no means easy, nor was it quick. Years. Years of therapy and peeling away the lies and fear and trauma, then piecing me back together with and in truth and love and healing.

The sponsor, the doctor and the pastor would talk quite regularly and keep each other abreast of my progress, struggles and goals. They each played a vital position in the team that the Lord had assembled. As I look back - no one was on the bench! Ever! Even a lot of "pinch hitting" for each other in those early days.

The family that had originally taken me in was part of the prayer team, the pastors, some of the elders of the church, several women known to be women of the Word and prayer, and a few men also-prayer warriors and lovers of God and His Word. They would meet with me some Sunday mornings before service and I believe other times during the week if necessary. I am sure that each of them prayed daily and throughout the day, sought the wisdom of His Spirit and His Word continuously personally and for one another as well.

Lifting up one another to the Throne of The Father and crying out for Him to work ~ revealing truth, protection, freedom, strength, wisdom, and healing.

This is definitely the part that I can only speak of what I remember and what the Lord did on my behalf from my point of view. The others that were involved in the process have their own views, memories and victories. As I have noted previously, I am unable to recall all that transpired in those years.

The pastor of family life and counseling (he had a master's in counseling as well as his divinity degree and was an ordained minister) was also a friend of the sponsor and their extended family. So, they often would encourage each other and help each other understand some of the clinical issues.

Their commitment to the Lord and helping me along this healing journey deserves (in my estimation) far beyond a medal of valor or a Purple Heart! All of them even went as far as driving halfway across the country to go to a conference to learn more about what I was dealing with and how best to help. That is a true picture of mission to the lost and dying within our midst in the local Body of Christ. It must be resurrected and only can be as we die to self and live for Him and the Father's work in and through each of us for His Kingdom!

What I felt during that time was a mixture of extreme

terror, anger, lack of control and helplessness. I was losing it mentally and could not remember several whole days. While I was working, I often would sketch to pass the time at the front desk of the workout facility. That was a wonderful gift of freedom and release for me. I sketched a picture of Jesus reaching out too little kids playing around a middle eastern home. There was one just out of reach and one looking on from behind Him. He was calling to them to come to Him. I noted the verse on the back of the sketch

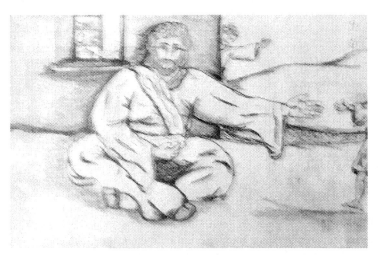

Figure 9- He calls to the little ones!

LUKE 18:16 (NLT)

"Then Jesus called for the children and said to the disciples, "Let the children come to me. Do not stop them! For the Kingdom of God belongs to those who are like these children."

I felt inside very much like I could hear Him calling to me to come and let Him care for me, but afraid of Him all at the same time.

That day during a counseling session with the Pastor, it was figured out that I had developed in my early childhood something they call "disassociation". Each long period of trauma caused a piece of my mind as it were to split off and contain itself in that age and those memories and characteristics. I do not know all the clinical terms for it or how it happens exactly. I am not a neuroscientist nor a Doctor of Psychology and complex trauma. Some people know this as multiple personality disorder/ disassociation identity disorder. This can be healed, despite what some clinicians say or have experienced. With the hand of our all-powerful Jehovah Rapha and experienced complex trauma specialist, along with a number of willing, wise servants I can type this as one whole, healed mind. It would take literally more than a decade of intense therapy and consistent vigilance in repetitive truth speaking to get to this beautifully free whole state.... but He is patient with us and love us too much to leave us shattered and in darkness. He makes the impossible-possible!

A REFRESHER ON DISASSOCIATION

When abuse first began and continued through my late teens those times were trapped in different parts of my brain. It is like when you separate out coins in separate containers just their sizes. The terror dreams, flashbacks, lost days and extreme anxiety were all symptoms that the shattered brain was breaking open, kind of spilling over sideways on all fronts. Why it happened at this time I do not know. Other than the Lord is Sovereign and had purposed these works for His children to do in Him from before the creation of the world.

> ### EPHESIANS 2:10 (NLT)
> *"For we are GOD's masterpiece. HE has created us anew in Christ Jesus, so we can do the good things He planned for us long ago."*

I was overwhelmed and fearful because of what happened in college the last time they thought I was suicidal and put me on that psych floor. I wanted to run when the doctor said what the pastor had discerned, and she had confirmed by several symptomatic factors. I did not want this to be true of me! Why would these recurring dreams, flashbacks, and other manifestations of evil just not go away and leave me in peace and wholeness? Wasn't there something simple that I could do to make it all stop and couldn't I just buck up and be okay with it all? Apparently not.

She began shedding light on all that had happened in my childhood. Trauma was carefully addressed and looked at and spoken out, walking through each piece that I could muster up to address with the doctor, who spoke truth and wisdom to it, in gentle yet firm steps. Lies, that I had lived under the power of, their impregnable stronghold, were revealed and destroyed individually by the power of Jesus Name and scripture. These scriptures were then read repeatedly in light of any thought that was contrary to that scripture.

TRUTH STRIKES A DEATH BLOW TO LIES

His Word is life! These wonderfully powerful truths were memorized and built up into a fortress that was stronger and greater than the ruins of lies! His Word is living and active. There is a reason He calls us to take every thought captive.

2 CORINTHIANS 10:5 (NIV)
"We demolish arguments and every pretension that sets itself up against the knowledge of GOD, and we take captive every thought to make it obedient to CHRIST."

For if we do not take them captive, they may take us captive and make us a slaves, and when a lie of the enemy of our souls makes us a slave, that journey it will set us on will only lead us in a path away from Christ Jesus-never toward Him. So be free, by freeing your mind of lies and thinking that is contrary to His Spirit and His Word. We need one another to encourage us in this process. That is why He says to encourage each other daily with these truths, and even more as we see the day of His return approaching.

I THESSALONIANS 5:11(NIV)
"Therefore, encourage each other and build each other up, just as in fact you are doing."

HEBREWS 10:25 (NIV)
"Do not give up meeting together, as some are in the habit of doing, but encourage one another–and all the more as you the Day approaching."

Jesus proclaimed He was the One that was prophesied to DO just that- to set captives free. He is still the One Who sets us free. He has the power to free us from destructive thoughts and stop us from sitting in the prison of depression and fear!

LUKE 4:17-19 (NLT)
"The scroll of the prophet Isaiah was handed to Him (Jesus). He unrolled the scroll and found the place where this was written: 'The Spirit of the Lord is upon me, for He has anointed me to bring Good News to the poor. He has sent Me to proclaim freedom to the captives and recovery of sight to the blind, to set the oppressed free, to proclaim the year of the Lord's favor"

I am one of many that Jesus the Son of God has set free. When He does this work for us, then we are really free indeed! In my Father's house there is a place for me now and I hold fast to that truth and sure hope. It gets me through the days after a memory that has tried to handcuff me in the night. The fact that I am a child of the Living God changes my destiny forever. It rings true in the song that proclaims the very fact that we are chosen not forsaken, we are exactly who He says we are, not what someone has labeled us or we ourselves. This song repeats often in my head these days. It is a faithful reminder of who I really am. Listening to songs that speak truth is one way to take those thoughts captive and destroy their power. It is a lie that can be powerful, the lie of being worthless, damaged, shattered pieces of refuse-unloved, unwanted and without hope. They are all lies that must be demolished by truth!

JOHN 8:36 (ESV)
"So, if the Son sets you free, you will be free indeed."

When we mentally become separated from JESUS through thoughts that are overpowering or fear, then just like sheep- our brains get caught in all kinds of brambles and may even walk right off a cliff to our demise. Lies and trauma seek to separate us from the only One Who can lead us to safety and healing.

So, scripture and music that speaks scripture and exalts and praises The Lord are a vital tool in the healing of the mind. They were essential in my healing. They will continue to be vital in my life and daily bread until I die!

The tape that the doctor had made to help me was full of scripture that spoke specifically to the lies and trauma I was fighting to overcome. This was an invaluable positive exercise for my brain and a healing balm. Today it would be akin to making a playlist on your streaming media device. We are continually being shaped by the thoughts we entertain in our minds. Whether good or bad. We either create new healthy cells by positive truthful thoughts or destroy cells through negative hopeless stressful ones.

PROVERBS 23:7 (AMPLIFIED VERSION)
"For as a man thinks in his heart, so is he."

Actions come out of thoughts. Our mind is an amazing thing. So, we are encouraged to have the mind of Christ. This is what they were all working toward in me. They were like Jesus, Paul, Barnabas and even Peter at times in his boldness. Replacing the old with the new. In various forms and through every day. I longed to be whole and well and at peace. It was if every moment of every day I fought a very real war within. There was only One who could completely heal my mind and fill me with hope for a better tomorrow. That was Jesus Himself. He did that often. Through song, His Word, dreams that were of Him and His return and very real fighting for me. He was fighting for me. He loved me. He loved me through those people, He loved me through His Word, He loved me through His praises that brought peace and calmness to my broken sprit and mind.

I CORINTHIANS 2:10-15
"We can resist temptations and pride as we stand with Him."

He was profoundly changing me day by day. His voice was becoming clearer the freer that I became. It is a continual process. With it becoming day by day clearer and so much stronger than the lies, trauma, or other harmful human voices that caused fear and shutting down. Healing was overcoming those wounds that had festered to an almost fatal state, because they had been gaping open within, yet hidden, deep and full of sickness. Jehovah Raphe (The God Who Heals) was actively healing me. I was and am deeply grateful for His mercy and grace that He would lavish on this nobody from nowhere.

The process is well worth the outcome. Being made whole in mind, in Spirit and in body. Some things need to be completely cutoff, torn down, broken, and or cast off in order for us to transform and be conformed more and more into His image. All those parts, mind-body-spirit, were extremely sick, shattered and decaying rapidly before. Now they were being put back together by His Mighty and Faithful hands through the work of His Holy Spirit, His servants, His Word, He Himself!

What the enemy of our souls and those who follow after his ways, meant for evil and perverseness-God the Father and Creator of my every cell - has been transformed for His glory and my good. My heart cries out in praise daily for all that He has done. Oft times we need only stay still and He Himself fights for us; other times we need to engage with Him in the battle and do our part in being obedient to His Word and walking in faith through the valleys and deep waters and fire at times. Knowing He is Faithful to bring us through.

Isaiah 43:2-3(ESV)
"When you pass through the waters, I WILL BE WITH YOU; and through the rivers, they shall not overflow you. When you walk through the fire, you shall not be burned, nor shall the flame scorch you. For I am the Lord your God, the Holy One of Israel, you Savior."

Psalm 23:4 (NLT)
"Even though I walk through the valley of the shadow of death, I will fear no evil; for YOU ARE with me; Your rod and Your staff, they comfort me.

2 Chronicles 20:17 (NLT)
"But you will not even need to fight. Take your positions; then stand still and watch the LORD's victory!"

1 Peter 1:6-7 (NLT)
"So be truly glad. There is a wonderful joy ahead, even though you must endure many trials for a little while. These trials will show that your faith is genuine. It is being tested as fire tests and purifies gold. So, when your faith remains strong through many trials, it will

*bring you much praise and glory and honor on the day
when Jesus Christ is revealed to the whole world"*

He is still Holy no matter what, and He is our defender! Not just for me-for all eternity, it is He Who is, was and always will be SOVEREIGN and our Great Defender.

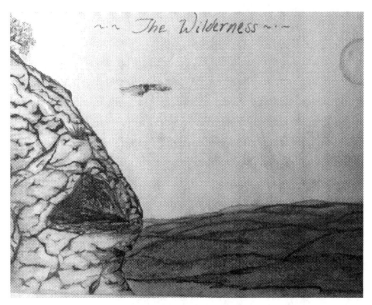

Figure 10- In the Wilderness of Life

Be still in the wilderness of waiting and pain, simply worship HIM in Spirit and truth and you will experience the sound of His voice of strength for another day.

CHAPTER **16**
THE VOICE OF THE LORD

PSALM 29: 1-11 (New Living Translation)
«Honor the Lord, you heavenly beings; honor the Lord for his glory and strength. Honor the Lord for the glory of his name. Worship the Lord in the splendor of his holiness.

The voice of the Lord echoes above the sea. The God of glory thunders. The Lord thunders over the mighty sea.

The voice of the Lord is powerful.

The voice of the Lord is majestic.

The voice of the Lord splits the mighty cedars; the Lord shatters the cedars of Lebanon. He makes Lebanon's mountains skip like a calf; he makes Mount Hermon leap like a young wild ox.

The voice of the Lord strikes with bolts of lightning.

The voice of the Lord makes the barren wilderness quake; the Lord shakes the wilderness of Kadesh.

The voice of the Lord twists mighty oaks and strips the forests bare. In his Temple everyone shouts, "Glory!" The Lord rules over the floodwaters. The Lord reigns as king forever.

The Lord gives his people strength. The Lord blesses them with peace."

~~~ 7 times "The voice of the LORD" is repeated...

When the number seven is used in scripture it is exemplifying completeness, perfection or finality. In this particular Psalm written by Israel's King David, he declares seven different attributes or actions of THE VOICE OF THE LORD and in doing so, he firmly states that it is perfect, complete and final! This is The VOICE of God Himself and it is the same voice that speaks today. Listen for it carefully and you too will hear it. The breath of God is still filled with power and healing.

His voice is the one that heals even the most shattered mind; it is the voice that calls out to the lost soul, the voice that whispers truths that can destroy all the lies of the enemy and it is the same voice that gives life and strength and peace to His children even today at this very moment that you are reading, He is speaking. Be still, wait patiently, seek expectantly and know He is calling out in love to each one who has ears to hear. He inclines His ear to hear our cries...oh that we would do the same to hear His voice answering and restoring.

Healing is available. The process will only come to fruition in His time and perfect plan if the broken one is willing to trust the One Who formed them and those who follow Him and His perfect Word, and then to believe and obey The Voice of the LORD above all others.

He has healed me physically and emotionally, mentally and

spiritually. HE IS THE GREAT PHYSICIAN; HE ALONE IS OUR TRUE HEALER!

I was physically very ill and it rendered me unable to walk often. I would wear a brace for years because of a neurological illness that caused drop foot and a gait dysfunction. But now I walk without a brace or cane or walker or any other aid because He graciously healed my drop foot that the doctors said cannot be healed. He did this at the same time He gave me a gift of the Holy Spirit - while I was at His altar praying for another. He gives good gifts, even when we do not specifically ask for them. May we not ever limit His great power and grace! He has been so powerful and gracious on my behalf my in healing me over and over when everyone else had acquiesced.

I am a grateful REFUGEE and wholly REDEEMED one in Christ Jesus...and more than a conqueror: A VICTOR and I walk in victory as I hold fast to His footsteps and look to His face and His Spirit within that guards my heart and mind and empowers me for each new day. No longer under a curse or condemnation, no longer walking in darkness being tormented by those that live in the shadows, no longer a slave to evil, no longer separated from The Voice of the LORD! Praise His Holy Name!!!

PSALM 91:1-16 (NIV)

"He who dwells in the shelter of the Most High will abide in the shadow of the Almighty. I will say to the Lord, "My refuge and my fortress, my God, in whom I trust." For he will deliver you from the snare of the fowler and from the deadly pestilence. He will cover you with his pinions, and under his wings you will find refuge; his faithfulness is a shield and buckler. You will not fear the terror of the night, nor the arrow that flies by day, nor the pestilence that stalks in darkness, nor the destruction that wastes at noonday. A thousand may fall at your side, ten

thousand at your right hand, but it will not come near you. You will only look with your eyes and see the recompense of the wicked. Because you have made the Lord your dwelling place— the Most High, who is my refuge— no evil shall be allowed to befall you, no plague come near your tent. For he will command his angels concerning you to guard you in all your ways. On their hands they will bear you up, lest you strike your foot against a stone. You will tread on the lion and the adder; the young lion and the serpent you will trample underfoot. "Because he holds fast to me in love, I will deliver him; I will protect him, because he knows my name. When he calls to me, I will answer him; I will be with him in trouble; I will rescue him and honor him. With long life I will satisfy him and show him my salvation."

Romans 8:1-13, 15-39 ESV

"There is therefore now no condemnation for those who are in Christ Jesus. For the law of the Spirit of life has set you free in Christ Jesus from the law of sin and death. For God has done what the law, weakened by the flesh, could not do. By sending his own Son in the likeness of sinful flesh and for sin, he condemned sin in the flesh, in order that the righteous requirement of the law might be fulfilled in us, who walk not according to the flesh but according to the Spirit. For those who live according to the flesh set their minds on the things of the flesh, but those who live according to the Spirit set their minds on the things of the Spirit. For to set the mind on the flesh is death, but to set the mind on the Spirit is life and peace. For the mind that is set on the flesh is hostile to God, for it does not submit to God's law; indeed, it cannot. Those who are

in the flesh cannot please God. You, however, are not in the flesh but in the Spirit, if in fact the Spirit of God dwells in you. Anyone who does not have the Spirit of Christ does not belong to him. But if Christ is in you, although the body is dead because of sin, the Spirit is life because of righteousness. If the Spirit of him who raised Jesus from the dead dwells in you, he who raised Christ Jesus from the dead will also give life to your mortal bodies through his Spirit who dwells in you. So then, brothers, we are debtors, not to the flesh, to live according to the flesh. For if you live according to the flesh you will die, but if by the Spirit you put to death the deeds of the body, you will live.

For you did not receive the spirit of slavery to fall back into fear, but you have received the Spirit of adoption as sons, by whom we cry, "Abba! Father!" The Spirit himself bears witness with our spirit that we are children of God, and if children, then heirs—heirs of God and fellow heirs with Christ, provided we suffer with him in order that we may also be glorified with him. For I consider that the sufferings of this present time are not worth comparing with the glory that is to be revealed to us. For the creation waits with eager longing for the revealing of the sons of God. For the creation was subjected to futility, not willingly, but because of him who subjected it, in hope that the creation itself will be set free from its bondage to corruption and obtain the freedom of the glory of the children of God. For we know that the whole creation has been groaning together in the pains of childbirth until now. And not only the creation, but we ourselves, who have the first fruits of the Spirit, groan inwardly as we wait eagerly for adoption as sons, the redemption of our bodies. For in this hope we were saved. Now hope that is seen is not hope. For who hopes for what he sees? But if we hope for what we do not see, we wait for it with patience. Likewise, the Spirit helps us in our weakness. For we do not know what to pray for as we ought, but the Spirit himself intercedes for us with groaning too deep for words. And he who searches hearts knows what the mind of the Spirit is, because the Spirit intercedes for the saints according to the will of God. And we know that for those who love God all things work together for good, for those who are called according to his purpose. For those whom he foreknew he also predestined to be conformed to the image of his Son, in order that he might be the firstborn among many brothers. And those whom he predestined he also called, and those whom he called he also justified, and those whom he justified he also glorified. What then shall we say to these things? If God is for us, who can be against us? He who did not spare his own Son but gave him up for us all, how will he not also with him graciously give us all things? Who shall bring any charge against God's elect? It is God who justifies. Who is to condemn? Christ Jesus is the one who died—more than that, who was raised—who is at the right hand of God, who indeed is interceding for us. Who shall separate us from the love of Christ? Shall tribulation, or distress, or persecution, or famine, or nakedness, or danger, or sword? As it is written, "For your sake we are being killed all day long; we are regarded as sheep to be slaughtered." No, in all these things we are more than conquerors through him who loved us. For I am sure that neither death nor life, nor angels nor rulers, nor things present nor things to come, nor powers, nor height nor depth, nor anything else in all creation, will be able to separate us from the love of God in Christ Jesus our Lord."

His voice needs to speak on every aspect of life, and He does speak. To have ears that hear as well as a heart to obey and not fear is key. When I fail to allow it to be primary in my life, or fear human disapproval and failing, more than walking in what He calls me to-then I reap all the consequences of those actions. I am not condemned by Him. No. He has called us to Himself and to faith-it is a moment by moment obedience and His forgiveness and grace is great for the times that I still fail. There are just consequences. But nothing HE has done in me or my soul- can ever be undone!

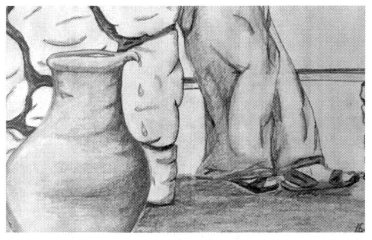

Figure 7- He knows everything about me!

CHAPTER 17

VOICES OF MARRIAGE

L ife after being made whole and translated from the kingdom of darkness to the kingdom of light was filled with encouragement and reassurance from both those who walked with me. The sphere of those who walked or persistently pressed through the long process of deliverance from the hand and hold of the enemy, to my physical healing as well as my new spiritual family was an ever expanding and morphing one.

After I was going through the extremely painful and long process of being made whole and spiritually free in mind and soul; there still were new avenues of trust to tread. There still are honestly. I was now engaged to that man the Lord had clearly told me his name years before, even while still in the throes of trying to break free from the hold of the valley and the darkness that had consumed my childhood, body, heart, soul and mind. The upcoming years would soon reveal all the physical damage cellular damage done by ongoing early complex trauma. Mentally and emotionally the first hurdles were about to be leapt into.

We were good friends for a year and a half and then married after a year and a half of premarital counseling from both the doctor and our then pastor, who also counseled both myself and then us as a couple. When the pastor gave us a questionnaire at the end of his portion of counseling, he said that we were the most prepared couple he had ever counseled and the best fit that he had seen God put together. That was an encouraging way to start life together, especially with my background.

Because of the abuse that I had endured and some other complicated health issues, the doctors had told us that we would not be able to have children without medical intervention. That was fine with both of us, as I was in no way wanting to be a parent nor did I feel in the least bit qualified for such a responsibility. I was sure I would mess them up and had no idea how to even change a diaper. He was more than thankful, because he traveled 60% of the time for work and wanted to continue to build up his savings and do what he wanted to do when he wanted to do it.

Life began fairly well in the first couple months; we had gone on a belated extensive honeymoon through the Canadian Rockies and traveled to Colorado for him to speak at a university there then hiking in the Canadian Rockies. It all seemed quite idyllic.

Then one day he came home from a trip and there was an issue with the apartment toilet, and he got terribly angry and began throwing things out the door and yelling. In response, I shut down and curled up in the corner of the kitchen behind a chair so that he would not hurt me. I had never ever seen this side of him. We had been friends for a year and a half before we began dating and then got engaged. So, I had known him for three years and had never experienced any outbursts of anger or even raising of his voice prior to this incident. Fear encapsulated me once again.

I would need to make a choice. I called my sponsor and she talked to both of us and explained my response to his anger and gave him some pointers on expressing it without such explosive actions. She also reminded me of truth and of who he was and that she believed I was safe and to pray and she would be praying too. One of a hundred or more times I would seek her counsel and discernment.

We both worked and enjoyed working and helping at the

"fam's" home with outdoor projects and the family home in the mountains. This was the same family that took me in and so the routine of getting together often and working and playing alongside one another continued and we were now a part of that as a couple. He was involved with a small men's group at church and being discipled in the Word.

This was a great thing. There were 5 men that met regularly, and all the wives really got along well. This was unbelievable. They were quite a blessing to us as a young married couple. They had all been married for a long while and we were just starting out. They would come to be a source of wisdom, laughter and tears in the years to come.

As time went by, we were both in a routine of work, church, family and us. He had his travel and his men's group and the gym still and I had the family, counseling and bible study. The prayer team was still there and would continue to be throughout the years.

The Lord knew what HE had purposed for the next years... it would not be anything like what I had expected. But, would reveal again and again that HE is Lord and He is far beyond what we can think or imagine. He reveals His faithfulness and mighty power in every aspect of life. We just need to ask for eyes to see, ears to hear and hearts to understand.

As in everyone's life things come around corners unexpectedly and we are not prepared for their impact. This came in the way of the possibility of a child. When confronted with this news I was terrified. Both hope and the very real possibility of being a parent, as well as the most likely course of loss and sorrow. He too was not prepared for this news or what that would mean to our way of life that had become routine and easy. This was soon to change and for the better and new voice would enter our world and be one of joy, love, trust, and inquisitiveness.

CHAPTER 18
VOICES OF A MIRACLE ~ CHILDREN

She entered the world with a long fight on an icy cold night. The room was literally packed with a cacophony of voices yelling at me to not give up, encouraging me to literally press through the pain and to push with all I had in me to be a vessel to bring a new life into this world for a new heritage. A beautiful new voice of redemption and hope!

She changed the routine; she chose to be awake and always looking forward instead of taking in the simple pleasure of rest and peace. She loved to hear classical music and the sound of her grandma's voices. She loved to be read to and to explore every nook and cranny. She started speaking every thought that came into her beautiful sweet, precious mind as early as 10 months. She had an ongoing dialogue with her imaginary friend who was a toy action figure she carried everywhere. Then it was as if a switch shut off at around 5 years old. Her words became few and all that wisdom and fresh insights into this world were only known to her and her Lord until she was persuaded to share.

SISTERS

Another priceless voice came into our lives three years after hers and she was ecstatic to have a baby sister! She would tell her stories and they would create a whole world of fictional characters that they made up with their baby dolls and stuffed animals. The stories would be a mix of daily life, Bible stories and their imaginations. I could listen to them go on with this all day without tiring of their sweet love for one another and spurring one another on to laughter and new ideas. They were balls of energy and after the second sweet voice I was to become extremely ill and life would change soon again.

They were and are in most ways' complete opposites in personality, but they were and are still the best of friends and true sisters that have each other's backs and love unconditionally. To watch them interact continues to make me just sit in awe. Look what the Lord has done! Look how He has redeemed and created beautiful masterpieces from broken shattered black ashes. His perfect love and powerful cleansing blood have destroyed the works of the enemy and He is making all things new in Him. He has the final say. He creates beauty from ashes.

The things that they have taught me go far beyond any book could do, other than the Bible. Sometimes they have no idea that their responses either cut me to the heart or fill my heart so full it would burst if another drop were added. They are almost grown young women now and I appreciate them more and more each day for their uniqueness and perspectives. They also are the only ones that can cause my heart to cry out with everything in me to the Father for their care and protection! That His mighty angels be in charge over their every step and surround them and carry them each moment of every day until He returns or takes them home! They are His first and foremost, and I am blessed beyond words to have the privilege and daunting responsibility of being their Mama. What an honor. I do not take it lightly and cherish every moment. Time is fleeting and precious. Their words are fewer and fewer the older they get. I must listen even more closely.

MOTTLED RASH TO PARALYSIS

As the first entered kindergarten I awoke one morning with a rash all over my body and a high fever. I went to step out of the shower and my left leg would not move. I had no feeling in that side and I knew something was very wrong, but I had two little girls to take care of. I did not have time to figure this out. Soon the voices of many new doctors and others would enter our life and with them and a new church plant, there came many more battles and an increasing darkness seemed to be creeping into our home. It had gained a foothold in my husband or had had one that I was unaware of and it soon would come to light at my next lowest and sickest point. This time I was whole, but not sure that I mentally, emotionally or physically could withstand this blow to our lives.

The girl's world was to spiral down at about the same age for my oldest, as when my father left. My heart was sick at this realization. I screamed out to the heaven lies, "NO!!!!!"! This was not supposed to happen to them, their home was never to be shattered, their Daddy was supposed to be the faithful, honest, upright, godly man that I had envisioned in him. What the next decade held was pits of despair, horrible truths revealed, loneliness, anger, brokenness, a hardening, and silence on many levels. I did not see how I could go on. I had nothing left in me to fight or even breathe.

But God is NOT SILENT! He is a loving, pursuing warrior of righteousness and redemption. He is victor and His voice overcome all others! Hallelujah! Over and over and over. His grace, Mercy, faithfulness, provision, perseverance, care, and healing were experienced in exponential ways in all our lives.

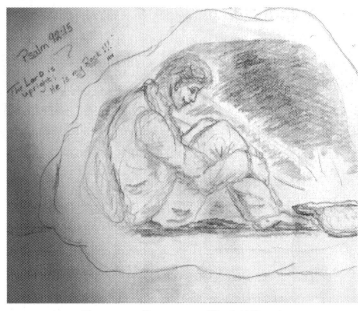

Figure 8- I am not a Rock! He is!

You are not the rock of refuge but you can hide in the Rock of Salvation and focus on Him and you will be safe and you will be strengthened for another day of fighting.

CHAPTER 19
VOICES OF DOCTORS
~ LIFE ALTERED & RESTORED

After a few weeks of progressively getting worse and seeing my immunologist/allergist and gastroenterologist as well as my primary. It was evident that they had no idea exactly what was happening, but it was as if it was the perfect storm of virus, weakened immunity, and something we would later find out to be a genetic mutation that caused my body to repeatedly get childhood diseases and have anaphylactic reactions to foods, medicines, chemicals, and venoms. It was called systemic mastocytosis, a rare and incurable disease that will end in leukemia.

By the fourth week after the high fever a friend had stopped in to drop off toys for the girls that her kids had grown out of and honestly to visually check on how I was physically doing. When I went to stand up from the couch I collapsed as my body was too weak to hold me up and I still had little to no feeling in the left leg and now the right foot was numb.

She insisted on taking me to the ER and I refused because the girls were at home and my husband was away on a trip for work, I could make do if she would just bring me a walker. My arms were strong enough I thought and I could carry myself and care for the girls that way.

She would not have any of that and said she was calling 911. I pleaded with her not to do that. The girls would be traumatized. I would call their grandmas and then I promised I would go to the hospital ER to get checked out.

That day turned into three weeks in the hospital with ever increasing numbness in my legs, arms, throat and face, they did several tests thinking it was Guion Barre syndrome, MS or some other neurological illness. They settled on several different theories. That small-town hospital sent me to a city hospital for testing and determined I had a virus on my brain stem. Also, they said the MS levels in my spinal fluid were on the higher side and I also had three lesions on my brain, although nothing was showing up in my neck or spine itself. Shortly after my release from acute rehab the then neurologist started treating me as if I had MS as well as now essential benign tremor. My head, voice, hands and legs tremored uncontrollably for months.

As the doctors were beginning to prepare me to go home, they came in my room and asked if everything was okay with my husband. I said that I think so. He is always steady and immovable. He never gets ruffled too much. They said that he seemed way to calm for the news they were going him. That they were not sure that he understood what my new condition would mean for our lives. So, they talked to him again, and he had the same calm response. That we would just live with it.

They sent me home in a wheelchair saying to get my house in order and that they had no idea how this would turn out but they had done all they could in the hospital and rehab. I was sent home in that wheelchair with a PT, OT and nurse. The house had been transformed on the main level with a ramp in the back and handicap accessories in the bathroom.

This was a time of extreme depression and fear. I did not know what even a moment held as I could no longer take care of myself or hold my sweet girls and read to them and take them to the lake and park and zoo. Our life as it was had truly ended. They were to suffer for no reason of their own because of a virus and my mutated genes' severe response. I had a rare disease called systemic mastocytosis as well as hypo gamma globular anemia. There were several other auto-immune issues that I dealt with and were most like exacerbated or stemmed from the very early onset of severe abuse.

I felt very overwhelmed and an all familiar voice rose inside of me saying there was no point to live. The girls and my husband would be far better off if I were dead and I began to ask the Lord to take me home. To supply a new godly wife for my husband and a caring, wise, loving mama for my beautiful gifts of daughters.

A DECADE ENDS IN FLAMES OF DECEIT

Those days were filled with being completely dependent on others for my food, bathing, dressing, and everything in between. Then on the day of our 10th anniversary the other shoe dropped! My husband was not who I thought and always proclaimed him to be. He was not faithful nor was he trustworthy.

I found out that he had been involved in the devastatingly dark world of homosexual pornography since High school and that he had gotten increasingly trapped in the addiction and lifestyle after we were married and he was one the road for work. He struggled with same sex attractions and he said that I had no idea how deep and dark it was and how far he had gone into this world.

This was like an atomic bomb to my already fragile brain and heart. I completely shut down. I was now not only numb physically but was again numb emotionally and spiritually at that moment. We were to go out for our anniversary to this nice restaurant and my family and best friend were on their way over to get me ready for the evening. When my best friend walked in, she felt it and say it on my face. She asked what had happened here?

The atmosphere of anger and disbelief was palatable. The

girls' grandma came and picked them up for their sleepover and they seemed none the wiser. For but a moment they did not have to face the reality of all that had transpired in the last few hours of that day and how our world had just imploded and what that would mean. Who knew the next 10 years would be one of continual struggle? In one way or another there was one battle after the next and my heart was once again guarded and continually distrusting.

Now I knew why he had not had a greater response in the hospital to my condition. That part of his brain was detached from feeling and numb as it were. With me in this condition he could live like he wanted to all the time, not just on the road. I was no longer a real homemaker/partner/wife, I was a disabled burden. I no longer felt like a wife or a mama at all or even a person. I felt like an object being moved around and trapped in a block of ice. The enemy loved this and I am sure was ready to end it all for all of us. I was not worth anything to anyone any longer and I had nothing to contribute to life...this was what played through my head from then on with louder and louder clarity. "You are nothing. You mean nothing. You are simply a burden and a waste. Be gone" were the phrases that turned over and over in my head night and day after that night.

A few weeks later when my husband left for a trip and they girls were at their grandmas and my friend was on her way over to check on me I laid out all my medicine on my bed and wondered if I should just take them all at once and go to sleep and never wake up again and everyone else would be better off.

The girl's "grandparents" were amazing and would raise them much better than I could ever and he could then live however he wanted for the rest of his days. The loud lies of the enemy were screeching these things over and over again in my ear and past failure and lack and not knowing if I would ever be able to take care of the girls or myself again was weighing on my heart like a lead weight!

That would have been a thoughtless and a permanent answer to a temporary situation and I am very thankful that the LORD absolutely intervened once again on my behalf. He has a way of thwarting our thoughtlessness! He had my "mom" from the family that took me in call me right at that moment. She asked what I was doing and she was on her way over to see me...I just broke down and wept and the next thing I knew she was sitting beside me on my bed. I had collapsed in tears and exhaustion on the floor beside the bed. I had slipped out of the wheelchair while sobbing. What was I to do? How could this be? How could he have deceived me and so many others this entire time. Some very godly, insightful, wise people. They were, that I was not. I certainly thought that we had covered everything possible with 13 months of premarital counseling.

Sometimes, you can never prepare for what you do not know.

We all were devastated and the same incredible support family and friends that had emerged as faithful and been girding us up through my illness were right there to speak truth and hope into the encroaching darkness of this almost fatal blow. It set me back in trust and love of anyone else immensely. It was as if I was again unlovable and of no worth. The difference from years before when this was the case was that I was now whole in mind and understood the consequences for the girls as well as myself more intensely than ever before. There was no escaping what the next months and years would hold for us.

They were to be ones of silence on my part, incredibly loneliness and protective Mama bear and self-preservation walls began to be firmly re-erected. I would withdraw and try to just live with the reality of being in a house with someone who was not the person I had thought I had married. He had disappeared along the ten-year journey, but I was completely physically, and financially dependent on him. I was once again trapped. I shut down. I allowed him to be passive aggressive and neglectful to me. But he was not permitted to neglect the girls, and he agreed to see this pastor from their school that did not know him, but dealt with this type of issues. He refused to see Dr. P or the pastor who counseled us.

After 8 months of living like this his parents came for their bi-annual visit. I was sitting in my wheelchair at the end of the ramp just staring at the ground when they arrived. I will never ever forget what they said to me. It was then and there that I knew that I could no longer live this lie. I could not do it. It was exhausting and making me even worse. The PT had said I had gone backwards and that because I was no longer showing forward improvement, they had to stop treatment. The OT had stopped coming months before.

That day I heard his voice tell me I would never walk without a walker and certainly never go upstairs every again in an almost condescending disappointed tone was the day I got angry! This anger was a healthy, I am done with this and what other people say, think and surmise about me, kind of anger.

We agreed to separate, and he would stay in town to be close to the girls. He was going to move far away with his parents at first so no one would interact with him. His parents said no. He had to take care of his daughters. The arrangements were drawn up and reviewed with and by Dr. P, my sponsor, himself, his counselor and myself. We met in Dr. P's office with the girls and the sponsor and he said that he had sinned against Mama and had to go to his own place to figure out things. So, a 10 ½ years after saying "I do" in great love and covenant before the Lord.... he moved out. It got noticeably quiet - yet again the journey was through a barren wilderness of loss.

God is one Who makes streams in the desert and life to spring up us of a wilderness. This time would be no different. After almost 7 years from that point on He miraculously healed my drop foot, overwhelmed me with His Holy Spirit in a way that I can never fully explain and set me completely free from my hatred and anger that entrapped me that day of our 10th anniversary announcement.

Jesus is my Hero and my continual Freedom Fighter! He is my life, my breath, my strength, my faithful Father and God! He alone is worth of all the praise of restoration of ruins that I had given up on and let just be a memorial to being cautious, guarded and wiser. Never to love another ever again.

Then He began to speak clearly during my morning quiet times with Him. From that moment at the altar when He baptized me with His Holy Spirit and gave me a wonderful gift, His Word became like a fresh new glass of water for this parched soul. Every word was alive, moving in my very life. Waking to a wooing to simply worship Him, seek Him, look for and find Him daily.

CHOKING, PNEUMONIA AND NO VOICE

Then one day I could not swallow right. I was choking on water. After a few days I choked on a piece of toast and started coughing uncontrollably until I heaved it all up. I was unaware that was a turning point for the next 3 years.

The Lord Himself cares for our needs in gracious and specific ways. The part of His Body that He had placed the girls and I in, by His grace and the prompting of my best friend, was a true life line of hope and encouragement and continuation of speaking life and truth into me over these next 7 years. And they continue to be more precious than I can express. The Lord is good, and the next trial would not be as hard as the previous. He had surrounded us once again, with a family of believers that cared for us in innumerable ways-both tangible and intangible.

This would usher in a second bout of severe pneumonia and upper respiratory infection with restrictive airway disease and vocal cord paralysis. Several stays in the hospital for 7-10days at a time and a new specialist in the city for vocal cords. I was rendered mute via my vocal cords that had stopped functioning properly and had somehow become paralyzed.

Once again, the specialists were baffled and now the video recording of my bronchoscopy is part of a research study. They had no idea how or why my throat and vocal cords were doing this; and it would take a specialist and vocal cord specialist and a team of other doctors to figure out how to get some of my voice back.

In the meantime, it would 6 mos. or more with absolutely no voice, and a severe cough. This turned into an incredibly special time that the Lord Himself literally pulled me in and whispered to me some priceless truths and promises and also some directions that were mind blowing.

HIS VOICE ONCE AGAIN OVERWHELMED ME AND I WAS CHANGED even in silence...His Whisper was like a trumpet to my ears. He is good! He is faithful! He has a plan and it is not the road that we think or imagine. His ways are higher and His thoughts far beyond what my mind could ever conceive. The best path is sometimes through the valley, to the other side into wide open spaces and new beginnings.

It was in this coming out of silence and learning to talk again through a vocal cord specialist and some amazing doctors in the city that I learned the value of breath. That breath and whispers are similar. You do not need your vocal cords to work properly to whisper. You just need breath. While at this point even my breath was limited due to acute severe persistent asthma that seemed to manifest out of nowhere. After much therapy and several times throughout each day, needing to do nebulizer medicinal breathing treatments my breathing and volume of air increased to a more normal volume. I went from only 27% lung function to 53% which felt like I was a new person. I could hold a conversation and walk without being winded or having a terrible coughing fit.

New life had come to my lungs and my heart was growing in grace and truth as His Spirit washed my mind and heart and soul with the water of His Holy Word.

The following February I was hit hard with the flu, my husband, who had three years earlier moved to the third floor of our home for financial reasons. He had made this his apartment which helped as the girls were going through the teenage years and hating to shuffle between home and his old apartment.

He stood at the foot of my bed and asked me to please forgive him for the destruction that he had caused to the girls lives as well as mine with his selfish acts. I told him that I had forgiven him in my mind, but at that moment my heart and soul fully forgave him, and restoration and healing began! Only God could do such a marvelous thing! Praise His Holy Name!

It was just like the apostle Paul told the Corinthian believers in his second letter to them:

2 Corinthians 5:18-19

"And all of this is a gift from GOD, who brought us back to Himself through Christ. And God has given us this task of reconciling people to Him. For God was in Christ, reconciling the world to Himself, no longer counting people's sins against them. And He gave us this wonderful message of reconciliation."

God was allowing me to experience this beautiful gift of forgiveness and reconciliation on a whole new level. It healed not only us, but something that seemed to weigh on our daughters as well. His Voice speaking peace and healing into our family once again and deeper still, was an immeasurable moment of divine love and compassion to His children.

I was feeling so much better and we went on our "first date" in 7 years and talked and His voice was sweet and honest and joyful. It was good to be together and learning afresh each other's new life. Then I began to cough.

This cough turned into a difficult to catch my breath kind of jag. The doctor happened to call to check on me and heard me as

I had just finished my breathing treatment and still could not take a deep breath. She told me to come to the office at once. They listened and both of my lower lobes were not moving any air. She gave me a shot of what she thought would help quickly open them up, but I happened to have an allergic reaction to it and then went into anaphylaxis as well.

Things moved quickly and they had me on oxygen and then an ambulance, lots of shots though intravenous lines and then the ER. Then quickly they moved me to telemetry and the medical floor with double pneumonia and tracheal bronchitis. I was extremely sick with a pneumonia that they said was not even from this area. They had no idea where I had picked it up. They called in another lung specialist and she evaluated me and changed the entire antibiotic and lung medicines regimen. In 24 hours, I began to breathe better. In the middle of the next night I began to react to the heparin shots, and they had to give my iv Benadryl. The hospitalist decided it would be safer if they could get me stable enough to go home on a strict antibiotic and lung treatment regimen with a Homecare nurse, occupational therapist and physical therapist as soon as possible. I was highly susceptible to secondary infection and the hospital was not the safest place for me to be. So, within three days they were able to stabilize me enough to return home with a team of clinicians to care for me.

I had gotten extremely weak and could hardly walk and lost a lot of weight. It took 4 months of care before I was back to walking and down to only two times a week physical therapy and neurology. The lung specialist confirmed that my systemic mastocytosis exacerbated my symptoms and made me terribly slow to heal from these setbacks. Thankfully, my church family and the family that took me in were all such priceless partners in my healing. Pastor said that a setback is just a great springboard for a great comeback! Our God is limitless and can do immeasurably more than all we ask or imagine! Ephesians 3:20-21 declares this truth.

By the end of August, I was feeling more like myself and made the trip to visit in-laws for the first time in ten years. It was a trip that would prove to be priceless as I was able to share the Word of God with my sister-in-law and give her a copy for her own to read for herself and prayed the Holy Spirit would make a way for her to know my Savior Jesus for herself. This is still my prayer for her to this day. He is faithful, I know His Word never returns to Him without carrying out all He has set it out to do. He is able to do a mighty work of healing and restoration if we will yield and patiently endure the process.

THE ENEMY ATTACKS WITH DISEASE

Upon returning my husband had his 50-year checkup. That night he ended up in the ER for the 3rd or 4th time in his entire life. He never gets sick and rarely goes to the doctor. But, after his colonoscopy he was in so much pain. He ended up having a cat scan to make sure they did not rupture anything. This too was a gift from the Lord. When the results of the scan came back to the ER doctor, she was very sober as she entered his bed area. The results showed he had 15 gallstones and she was not surprised he was in pain. They could take care of that simply the next couple of days in a routine surgery. It was Labor Day weekend, so the regular surgeon was not on. The surgeon on was the one who had done multiple of my surgeries and was a believer. Then she gave us the rest of the report.

The cat scan showed that he had a large mass on his right kidney. This type of mass is called renal cell carcinoma. He has kidney cancer. This type of cancer is profoundly serious and usually goes unnoticed until it is too far along for a good outcome. It has no symptoms until it has metastasized on the surrounding organs or in the lungs, brain or both kidneys. God had allowed him to consent to a 50-year checkup colonoscopy, to show the gallstones, to reveal the cancer before it had gone too far. Praise His Holy Name!

He had a partial nephrectomy 4 weeks after he had his gallbladder removed. His abdomen looked like he had been in a war and got hit with tons of shrapnel. 11 incisions and 2 infections later he was finally on the mend. Hallelujah.

About the time for his 3-month follow-up cat scan something came into the world that had stopped the world and our country's way of life as we had known it. Corona Virus 19, COVID-19 as they call it. A pandemic.

Many countries, including ours were under a governmental shelter where you are ordered to shelter in place. Only essential businesses were allowed to stay open and you were only permitted to leave your house if you were an essential worker or had to go to perform a life-sustaining function (i.e. medicine retrieval, groceries, doctor or hospital). This could have triggered more terror or a deep seeded fear of entrapment once again.

It did not. Because of the Lord's great love and repeated faithful deliverance of myself and my family, we are excited about what He will do in this time to bring many to Himself in salvation.

This is an unprecedented time for us and a wonderful opportunity to clearly hear the gospel over every possible media outlet as live-streaming is on-going of Bible Studies, encouragement, praise and worship and family devotions like never before. The gospel is going forth at an unheard-of pace! Hallelujah, hallelujah, hallelujah!

We are having a global call to prayer and repentance as the Body of Christ in response to God's call to us in 2 Chronicles 7:14 and Joel 2. The church corporately is petitioning God the Father to once again forgive us and heal us and set this world free from the effects of our blatant sin and turning away as a country from Him and His Word. May He once again soften hard hearts, give people an ear tuned to His voice and a longing for His will to be done on earth as it is in heaven.

His VOICE and Holy Spirit alone can again begin redeeming the years the locusts of business and distraction had eaten away from families and life in general!

He absolutely will redeem all things and make all things new one day.

> REVELATION 21:3-7 (NLT)
>
> *"I heard a loud shout from the throne, saying, "Look, God's home is now among his people! He will live with them, and they will be his people. God himself will be with them. 4He will wipe every tear from their eyes, and there will be no more death or sorrow or crying or pain. All these things are gone forever."*
> *5And the one sitting on the throne said, "Look, I am making everything new!" And then he said to me, "Write this down, for what I tell you is trustworthy and true." 6And he also said, "It is finished! I am the Alpha and the Omega—the Beginning and the End. To all who are thirsty I will give freely from the springs of the water of life. 7All who are victorious will inherit all these blessings, and I will be their God, and they will be my children."*

I know that I am just a drop in the ocean of redeemed lives in His sea of forgiveness and eternal love! I praise His Holy Name and will continue to do so for all eternity as His Voice gets clearer and clearer until it is the strong sound of RUSHING WATERS and TRUMPET BLASTS and we fall before Him in worship and unashamed adoration!! Saying here I am Lord to Worship YOU, you alone are worthy! You alone are Holy and Almighty! Yours is the Kingdom, the Power and the Glory forever and ever!

Therefore, until He comes, or takes us home may your ear turn to listen for His Voice. Then you will indeed find it truly is the VOICE of freedom and redemption along with a myriad of other wonderful things that will bring you a renewed hope and life like you have never experienced before you heard Him. His voice conquers all others and redeems all that this world and the enemy sought to steal from you. He is our REDEEMER and HEALER! Listen and be free and victorious!

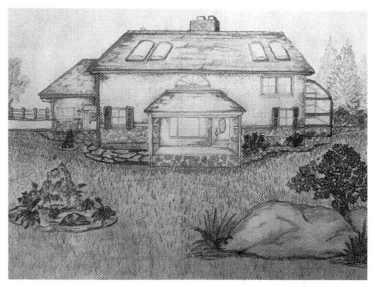

Figure 6-Dreaming of a Healthy Home

EPILOGUE

There are millions of children who are living through this kind of life and there are millions of adults out there who have endured the same upbringing or worse. They are hiding in fear of the threats that were spoken over and over to them if they ever told or they feel as though they are going out of their mind with anxiety with all the memories of the horrors that they endured.

The reason for this retelling is for each of them. The goal is that they will seek help and a safe place to deal with all these things in the presence of the Lord Jesus. That each one might know that they are not what their abusers said about them, they are an amazing creation of the Almighty Good Father. They have endured the effects of the evil and sins of others in horrific unimaginable ways and have survived! They have innocently been the carnage of this fallen and depraved generation in which we must now live. It is to them that I write this to encourage them that there is more to this life; much more that is good and worthy of your healing and steadfast perseverance toward that healing and to a life you were created for! A life that is more than you can dare imagine.

May each one come to know that there is a way out. There is a POWERFUL OVERCOMING Voice that you can trust and that loves individually and with a pure perfect love that will cast out all those lies and fears. This Redeemer will destroy the terror of the night and the attacks during the day. His name is Jesus! The Only Son of the Living God and He is the Way, the Truth and the Life!

Just like many before He WILL set each one that comes to Him free! It is a long, hard journey where there are more times than can be counted where the urge to quit amid the process will be strong.

Do not quit! Just keep going! It will be supremely worth it when that corner is turned, when the voices of the past are silenced and rendered powerless. When the Voice you hear is one of Eternal Hope and a Future of great things beyond our imaginations! Keep going and listening for life and light and truth. You will find Him if your truly seek Him. You will hear words of encouragement, wisdom and true love.

Ephesians 3:12-21 (NLT)

"Because of Christ and our faith in him, we can now come boldly and confidently into God's presence. So please do not lose heart because of my trials here. I am suffering for you, so you should feel honored. When I think of all this, I fall to my knees and pray to the Father,

"I pray that from His glorious, unlimited resources He will empower you with inner strength through his Spirit. Then Christ will make His home in your hearts as you trust in Him. Your roots will grow down into God's love and keep you strong. And may you have the power to understand, as all God's people should, how wide, how long, how high, and how deep His love is. May you experience the love of Christ, though it is too great to understand fully. Then you will be made complete with all the fullness of life and power that comes from God. Now all glory to God, who is able, through his mighty power at work within us, to accomplish infinitely more than we might ask or think. Glory to him in the church and in Christ Jesus through all generations forever and ever! Amen."

BIBLIOGRAPHY

Chapter 3

1   Lewis, C. (May 5, 1955). *THE MAGICIAN"S NEPHEW.* London,
    UNITED KINGDOM: The Bodley Head.

Printed in the United States
By Bookmasters